Gastric Cancer - Progress and Challenges in the Era of Precision Medicine

Edited by Daniela Cornelia Lazar

Published in London, United Kingdom

Gastric Cancer - Progress and Challenges in the Era of Precision Medicine
http://dx.doi.org/10.5772/intechopen.111116
Edited by Daniela Cornelia Lazar

Contributors
Ahmad Bello Kumo, Ali Ahmadi, Daniela Cornelia Lazăr, Eunji Jang, Jae-Ho Cheong, Javad Mohammadnejad, Josaphat Ndelo di Phanzu, Lievins-Corneille Mputu Malolo, Min-Kyue Shin, Patrick Ndelo Matondo, Pegah Mousavi, Seyed Mohammad Hosseini, Shakila Behzadifar, Yannick Belo Nuapia, Yong-Min Huh

First published in London, United Kingdom, 2024 by IntechOpen
IntechOpen is the global imprint of INTECHOPEN LIMITED, registered in England and Wales, registration number: 11086078, 167-169 Great Portland Street, London, W1W 5PF, United Kingdom

British Library Cataloguing-in-Publication Data
A catalogue record for this book is available from the British Library

Additional hard and PDF copies can be obtained from orders@intechopen.com

Gastric Cancer - Progress and Challenges in the Era of Precision Medicine
Edited by Daniela Cornelia Lazar
p. cm.
Print ISBN 978-0-85466-443-6
Online ISBN 978-0-85466-442-9
eBook (PDF) ISBN 978-0-85466-444-3

For EU product safety concerns:
IN TECH d.o.o., Prolaz Marije Krucifikse Kozulić 3, 51000 Rijeka, Croatia,
info@intechopen.com or visit our website at intechopen.com.

Meet the editor

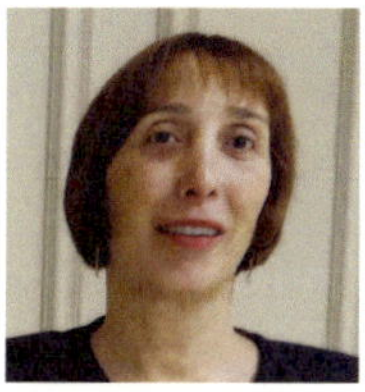

Associate Professor Dr. Daniela Lazar began her career in a center of excellence, the Department of Gastroenterology and Hepatology, University of Medicine and Pharmacy "Victor Babes," Timisoara, Romania, where she acquired clinical skills in gastroenterology, learned the techniques of endoscopy and abdominal ultrasonography and began her research activity. Besides gastroenterology, she showed interest in the oncological field and the research of gastrointestinal neoplastic conditions, especially gastric cancer. Dr. Lazar is specialized in gastroenterology, medical oncology, and internal medicine. Currently, besides academic and teaching activities, she is performing integrated clinical practice in the Department of Internal Medicine, Emergency Military Clinical Hospital, Timisoara. Dr. Lazar wrote her Ph.D. thesis in the field of gastric cancer. She has participated in many national and international congresses with research studies in the field of gastroenterology, internal medicine, and digestive oncology. She published research studies in many renowned international journals regarding angiogenesis, premalignant lesions, and prognostic factors in gastric cancer. Also, she published review articles regarding targeted treatments and immunotherapy in gastric cancer, as well as the impact of artificial intelligence in diagnosing premalignant or malignant esophageal and gastric conditions. She is also interested in aspects regarding the epidemiology, phenotypes, and treatment of inflammatory bowel diseases, being part of the national and international working groups in this domain. Associate Professor Dr. Daniela Lazar was the author or coauthor of several books and book chapters with different gastroenterological, oncological, and internal medicine topics for fellows and specialists in these fields, edited by national publishers, as well as the author of books designated for students. Moreover, Dr. Lazar wrote many book chapters and was the academic editor of several books edited by well-known international publishers. Dr. Lazar is a reviewer for many international journals.

Contents

Preface

Gastric cancer, a formidable challenge in oncology, has persisted as one of the most lethal malignancies worldwide. Despite significant advances in understanding its pathogenesis and risk factors, the global burden of this disease remains alarmingly high. With the advent of precision medicine, there is renewed hope in the fight against gastric cancer—a hope rooted in the promise of tailoring treatment to the individual patient based on genetic, environmental, and lifestyle factors.

The geographic variability in the incidence of gastric cancer highlights the profound influence of environmental and lifestyle factors. Countries like Japan, Korea, and regions of Eastern Europe report the highest rates, whereas North America and much of Africa see lower incidences. This variability suggests that while genetic predisposition plays a role, modifiable factors such as diet and *Helicobacter pylori* infection are crucial determinants of disease risk. The advent of modern refrigeration, improvements in food preservation, and economic development have contributed to a decline in incidence and mortality in many parts of the world. However, the rise of diffuse gastric cancer in younger populations, particularly in the West, raises new concerns and questions that demand further exploration.

Helicobacter pylori, a once controversial agent in the etiology of gastric cancer, is now firmly established as a major modifiable risk factor. This bacterium, along with high-salt diets and the consumption of smoked and processed meats, underscores the importance of dietary influences on cancer risk. The epidemiological patterns observed across different populations illuminate the critical intersection of diet, infection, and cancer. As we delve deeper into the complex interplay of these factors, the importance of early detection and intervention becomes increasingly apparent. In regions like Japan and Korea, where endoscopic screening is routine, early-stage diagnosis has dramatically improved survival rates, showcasing the potential impact of early detection on disease outcomes.

The narrative of gastric cancer is also evolving with the introduction of innovative therapies. Immunotherapy, for instance, has opened new frontiers, offering hope where conventional treatments have often failed. By harnessing the body's immune system to combat cancer, this approach represents a paradigm shift in oncology. Alongside immunotherapy, the emergence of precision medicine—driven by advances in molecular subtyping and the identification of genetic markers—promises to revolutionize the management of gastric cancer. These developments underscore the necessity of integrating cutting-edge research into clinical practice to improve prognoses and extend survival.

This book, *Gastric Cancer – Progress and Challenges in the Era of Precision Medicine*, embarks on a comprehensive exploration of the multifaceted aspects of gastric cancer. From examining the pivotal roles of diet and *Helicobacter pylori* as modifiable risk factors to delving into the transformative potential of immunotherapy and precision medicine, this work seeks to illuminate the path forward in combating this deadly disease. As we navigate through the complexities of gastric cancer, the chapters within provide a detailed account of the current scientific understanding, innovative treatment strategies, and ongoing challenges that continue to shape this field.

The goal of this compilation is not merely to present the state of the art but to inspire a future where precision medicine becomes the cornerstone of gastric cancer treatment—where each patient's unique profile guides the therapeutic approach, leading to better outcomes and, ultimately, saving lives. As researchers, clinicians, and policymakers, we are called to collaborate in this endeavor, ensuring that the strides made in research translate into real-world benefits for those affected by this challenging disease.

Dr. Daniela Cornelia Lazăr
Associate Professor,
Department V of Internal Medicine I, Discipline of Internal Medicine IV,
University of Medicine and Pharmacy "Victor Babeş",
Timişoara, Romania

Section 1

Risk Factors and Toxicological Aspects of *H. pylori* Infection

Chapter 1

Introductory Chapter: An Updated Overview of Gastric Cancer

Daniela Cornelia Lazăr

1. Introduction

Despite a decreasing trend in incidence and mortality rates observed in the past few decades in numerous regions of the world, gastric cancer (CG) remains the fifth most common neoplasia and ranks the fourth place of cancer-related mortality overall. According to GLOBOCAN estimates, GC was responsible for over 1 million new cancer cases and three-quarters of a million deaths in 2020 globally. Also, it has been described a significant geographical variation in GC burden, with areas such as Asia where it remains severe, and several developing regions where an upward trend in both GC incidence and mortality rates is reported. These data highlight the fact that gastric cancer still represents a major health concern worldwide.

GC defines a primary tumor derived from the epithelial gastric lineage, gastric carcinogenesis being regarded as a multistep process, associated with several risk factors. Chronic H. Pylori (H.p) infection represents the major risk factor for the development of gastric cancer. H.p is a gram-negative spiral-shaped bacteria that infects more than 50% of world's population, classified by World Health Organization as a class one carcinogen for GC; it is responsible for approximately 90% of non-cardial cases of gastric tumors. Besides H. pylori, other gastric microbiota is correlated with the development of GC. Dietary and lifestyle factors such as lower intake of fruit/vegetables, higher intake of salt, salted, and processed food, as well as tobacco and alcohol consumption are demonstrated risk factors for GC. Other risk factors have been also described, including previous gastric surgery, pernicious anemia, the existence of a first-degree family member with GC, and several inherited cancer syndromes related to GC development, the strongest association being demonstrated in case of hereditary diffuse gastric cancer (CDH1) syndrome. According to the proximal *vs.* distal gastric location, GC is classified into cardia and non-cardia subtypes, the later accounting for more than 80% of GC cases globally. Gastric cardia tumors are more likely to be associated with Epstein–Barr virus (EBV) infection, diet, and higher BMI of the patient.

The most used classifications of GC are represented by the classical Lauren and the complex WHO pathohistological classification system, respectively. Currently, there are under investigation-specific GC signatures, encompassing the detection of human epidermal growth factor receptor 2 (HER2) expression, microsatellite instability, the presence of factors that regulate apoptosis, cell cycle or influence the properties of the cellular membrane, and presence of multidrug resistance proteins.

 IntechOpen

The classification performed in 2014 by Cancer Genome Atlas (TCGA) Research Network based on a complex molecular characterization of 295 untreated GC, categorized this neoplasia into four subtypes—MSI-H tumors, EBV (+) tumors, tumors exhibiting chromosomal instability (CIN), and genomically stable tumors. In the group of chromosomal instable cancers, receptor tyrosine kinases such as epidermal growth factor receptor (EGFR), fibroblast growth factor receptor (FGFR2), HER2, and also hepatocyte growth factor receptor (MET) are commonly overexpressed. Microsatellite instable and EBV-positive subtypes of GC often express immune checkpoint molecules such as ligand of programmed cell death 1 (PD-L1) and V-domain immunoglobulin (Ig)-containing suppressor of T-cell activation (VISTA), whereas genomically stable tumors exhibit alterations in claudin 18.2 expression. In advance tumors needing palliative treatment, next-generation sequencing techniques are nowadays frequently used to identify druggable targets. Nevertheless, due to intratumoral heterogeneity, most tissue-based biomarkers of GC are subjected to the risk of a sampling error; therefore, an accurate tissue specimen is essential.

Diagnostic tools for confirming and staging GC include upper endoscopy, histopathological, immunohistochemical and molecular characterization of the tumor, endoscopic ultrasound (EUS), CT scan of the chest, abdomen and pelvis, and also magnetic resonance imaging (MRI) and FDG-PET/CT scans for particular clinical indications, as well as surgical laparoscopy plus peritoneal cytology for identifying peritoneal carcinomatosis. In the initial assessment of GC patients with potentially resectable tumor, micro-satellite instability (MSI) testing at diagnosis may help deciding the best therapeutic strategy.

A multitude of factors have an impact on the prognosis of these patients, including patient-related factors such as gender, age and race/ethnicity, and tumor-related factors such as tumor's location, histological/molecular subtype, depth of invasion, presence of lymph node, and distant metastasis. Moreover, there are treatment-related factors with influence on patient's prognosis, different therapeutic approaches being developed according to the specific molecular characterization of the cancer—MSI-H/dMMR status, tumor mutation burden (TMB), HER 2 status, and PD-1 ligand (PD-L1) positivity—and stage of the tumor [1–4].

2. Targeted therapeutic algorithms and prevention strategies

Gastric cancer proved to be a heterogeneous tumor that needs a multidisciplinary approach for deciding the best therapeutic algorithm for a selected patient, encompassing specialties such as gastroenterology, pathology, radiology, as well as medical, radiation, and surgical oncology. Complex treatment strategies, including endoscopic resection in early cancers and surgical resection, neo-adjuvant and adjuvant chemotherapy, chemoradiotherapy, hyperthermic intraperitoneal chemotherapy (HIPEC), or pressurized intraperitoneal aerosol chemotherapy (PIPAC), as well as novel targeted treatments based on the molecular characteristics of the tumor, including multikinase inhibitors of angiogenic and oncogenic receptor tyrosine kinases (such as agents targeting VEGF receptors, HER2, and others), have been employed for the therapeutic management of gastric cancer patients. Despite the use of novel targeted agents, the survival benefice of these treatments remains limited in advanced and metastatic gastric cancers.

All the research and clinical data highlight the importance of the immune system in fighting against cancer development and progression. In this context, many immunotherapeutic strategies have been investigated, using monoclonal antibodies, cytokines, gene-transferred vaccines, cytotoxic cells, or T cells infusions in order to either increase the host antitumoral response, or the susceptibility to treatment of the tumor cells. In recent years, the therapeutic strategy and the outcome of many cancers, such as melanoma, non-small cell lung cancer (NSCLC), urothelial cell carcinoma, head and neck squamous cell carcinoma, Hodgkins lymphoma, and others changed fundamentally by introducing the immunotherapy, especially with implementation of treatment using immune checkpoints inhibitors, anti-cytotoxic T lymphocyte antigen-4 (CTLA-4) antibodies, and antagonists of the programmed death (PD)-1/PD-ligand 1 (PD-L1) pathway. Furthermore, there have been conducted several trials demonstrating a beneficial effect of immunotherapy used in different settings for gastric tumors, especially when administrated in highly selected subgroups of GC patients, who were considered as having good response criteria for this treatment. Also, there seems to be some promising results against GC when combining therapy of immune checkpoint inhibitors with other immunotherapies, targeted agents, and radio/chemotherapies, unfortunately at the expense of developing immune-related side effects.

Future directions in gastric cancer treatment include strategies targeting EGFR or agents targeting claudin18.2.

Due to the tumor heterogeneity, GC prevention necessitates a versatile approach, referring to an efficient implementation to H. pylori eradication guidelines, a more refined understanding of the determining factors of eradication failure and the most adequate attitude in this context, as well as improved guidelines to accurately detect and screen individuals having a high risk of progression across the premalignant stages of H. pylori-associated gastritis. Besides H.p eradication which has been demonstrated to be associated with a reduced risk of developing GC, endoscopic surveillance in individuals at increased risk for GC represents an essential screening method for preventing GC. In high-incidence areas, implementation of mass endoscopic surveillance programs was associated with reduces rates of GC incidence and mortality.

Novel predictive noninvasive circulating biomarkers for GC represent a modern approach to identify individuals at the highest risk of progressing toward this type of tumor, some of them already having a well-defined role in the clinical setting in some high-incidence areas. Moreover, liquid biopsy (detection of circulating tumor DNA) is emerging as a tool for GC diagnosis, therapy, and real-time surveillance. Another promising strategy for a better risk stratification of patients who are likely to develop GC is represented by genetic testing that offers a more personalized approach; in the future, increased accessibility to these tests and to an accurate clinical decision-making of all the tested patients will be needed [5–7].

In conclusion, we are witnessing a rapid development of advanced endoscopic devices and imaging techniques, with the introduction of artificial intelligence for improving the detection of both preneoplastic and neoplastic gastric lesions. Moreover, the is an evolution in therapeutic methods, with improvement in endoscopic resection techniques including endoscopic mucosal resection (EMR) and submucosal dissection (ESD), use of minimally invasive surgery, and the discovery of innovative therapeutic approaches. Taking into consideration the well-known heterogeneity of GC tumors, in the era of personalized medicine, new investigational diagnostic and prognostic biomarkers for GC and identification of genetic profiles are needed for better cancer detection and characterization, selection of specific therapeutic algorithms targeted to different subgroups of CG patients in order to obtain a superior treatment response, and an improved overall survival.

Author details

Daniela Cornelia Lazăr
Department V of Internal Medicine I, Discipline of Internal Medicine IV,
University of Medicine and Pharmacy "Victor Babeş", Timişoara, Romania

*Address all correspondence to: lazar_daniela@yahoo.com

References

[1] Yang WJ, Zhao HP, Yu Y, Wang JH, Guo L, Liu JY, et al. Updates on global epidemiology, risk and prognostic factors of gastric cancer. World Journal of Gastroenterology. 2023;**29**(16):2452-2468. DOI: 10.3748/wjg.v29.i16.2452

[2] Sung H, Ferlay J, Siegel RL, Laversanne M, Soerjomataram I, Jemal A, et al. Global cancer statistics 2020: GLOBOCAN estimates of incidence and mortality worldwide for 36 cancers in 185 countries. CA: A Cancer Journal for Clinicians. 2021;**71**(3):209-249. DOI: 10.3322/caac.21660. Epub 2021 Feb 4

[3] Röcken C. Predictive biomarkers in gastric cancer. Journal of Cancer Research and Clinical Oncology. 2023;**149**(1):467-481. DOI: 10.1007/s00432-022-04408-0. Epub 2022 Oct 19

[4] Alagesan P, Goodwin JC, Garman KS, Epplein M. Cancer Progress and priorities: Gastric cancer. Cancer Epidemiology, Biomarkers and Prevention. 2023;**32**(4):473-486. DOI: 10.1158/1055-9965.EPI-22-0994

[5] Joshi SS, Badgwell BD. Current treatment and recent progress in gastric cancer. CA: A Cancer Journal for Clinicians. 2021;**71**(3):264-279. DOI: 10.3322/caac.21657. Epub 2021 Feb 16

[6] Eom SS, Choi W, Eom BW, Park SH, Kim SJ, Kim YI, et al. A comprehensive and comparative review of global gastric cancer treatment guidelines. Journal of Gastric Cancer. 2022;**22**(1):3-23. DOI: 10.5230/jgc.2022.22.e10. Epub 2022 Mar 31

[7] Machlowska J, Baj J, Sitarz M, Maciejewski R, Sitarz R. Gastric cancer: Epidemiology, risk factors, classification, genomic characteristics and treatment strategies. International Journal of Molecular Sciences. 2020;**21**(11):4012. DOI: 10.3390/ijms21114012

Chapter 2

Gastric Cancer: Diet and *Helicobacter pylori* as Major Modifiable Risk Factors

Ahmad Bello Kumo

Abstract

Gastric cancer is ranked as the sixth cancer worldwide and the fourth leading cause of cancer-related deaths. There exists marked geographic variation in the incidence of gastric cancer the world over, with the highest rates reported in Japan, Korea, and Eastern Europe. The gastric cancer highest incidence regions of the world are Eastern Asia, Europe, Central and South America, while North America, Australia, and Africa are considered low incidence areas. Sex differences exist in gastric cancer incidence, which is almost two-fold higher in males than females. There is a declining incidence and mortality of gastric cancer in most parts of the world which is attributed to improved food preservation and storage associated with the advent of the refrigerator, improved economic development, and screening for early detection of gastric cancer, particularly in high incidence areas. The etiology of gastric cancer is multifactorial—The two major factors implicated in the development of gastric cancer are: genetic (non-modifiable) and environmental (modifiable) risk factors such as *Helicobacter pylori*, high intake of salt, red meat, and smoked fish/meat, which lead to increased incidence of gastric cancer, while increased consumption of leafy vegetables and fruits are generally protective.

Keywords: gastric cancer, diet, *Helicobacter pylori*, modifiable factors, risk factors

1. Introduction

Noncommunicable diseases (NCDs) are a significant contributor to global deaths and cancers are noted as the leading cause among the NCDs. Although the incidence of gastric cancer has steadily declined over the past two decades, nonetheless in 2018 mortality rates remain high at more than 8% of deaths from cancer worldwide [1].

Gastric cancer is the fifth most common cancer after cancers of the female breast, lung, colon, rectum, and prostate, with more than two-thirds of gastric cancer occurring in the developing countries. It is the third most common cause of cancer-related death worldwide [1, 2]. According to Globocan, there were more than 1,033,701 new cases of gastric cancer with 782,685 (75.7%) deaths in 2018. The gastric cancer highest incidence regions of the world are Eastern Asia, Europe (Central & Eastern), and Central and South America, while North America, Australia, and Africa with the exception of Southern Africa are considered to be low incidence areas [1, 2]. Sex differences exist in gastric cancer incidence, which is almost two-fold higher in males than females. The sex difference suggests the protective effect of sex steroid hormones in gastric cancer pathogenesis [3]. Likewise, studies have shown that males have higher risks of *Helicobacter pylori* infection (a major risk factor of gastric cancer) than females, which may also lead to sex differences [3, 4].

There is a decline in the incidence and mortality of gastric cancer in most parts of the developed world which is attributed to improved food preservation and storage associated with the advent of the refrigerator, improved economic development, and endoscopic screening for early detection of gastric cancer, particularly in high incidence areas like Japan, Korea, and China. Despite the declining rates of gastric cancer, recent evidence suggests that there are rising rates of diffuse type gastric cancer of the proximal stomach and rising incidence of gastric cancer in the young in the United States and the etiology of this rise may be multifactorial [5–9]. Over the past decades, there has been a change in the type and location of upper gastrointestinal tract tumors in North America and Europe, with a marked decline in intestinal type gastric cancers of the distal stomach in North America and Western European countries. This may be attributed to improved hygiene, modern food preservation, clean drinking water, drugs for *Helicobacter pylori* eradication, as well as dietary modification that promote low incidence of gastric cancer [8, 10–12].

The risk of gastric cancer rises steadily with advancing age, with the highest incidence rates occurring in the sixth and seventh decade of life, but rarely before the age of 50 years [5]. A study conducted over a 5-year period reported that 1.8% of gastric cancer cases occurred in individuals younger than 34 years, 38.6% in adults between 35 and 64 years old, and 59.6% occurred in elderly subjects over 65 years, with a median age at diagnosis of 68 years, indicating that gastric cancer risk increases with aging. In all populations, the age-standardized risk is about two to threefold higher in men than in women [13, 14].

In Africa, the rising incidence of gastric cancer was noted in the urban areas more than in the rural areas. The factors responsible for this rising incidence are increased awareness resulting from increased literacy levels, availability of diagnostic facilities, availability of specialist physicians/surgeons that aid early diagnosis, and westernization of diet from the proliferation of fast-food joints. It is noteworthy also to mention that patients diagnosed with gastric cancer in Africa are younger, mostly diagnosed in their third to fourth decade, and present at the late stage of the disease. Tijjani et al. reported the case of a 23-year-old woman presenting with severe bone pain as the first presentation who was found to have gastric cancer with bone metastasis [15]. The estimated incidence of gastric cancer in Africa is 4/100000 [16] and it was noted that at the time of diagnosis, metastatic diseases are predominant ranging from 50 to 78.6% of patients in the reported cases [16–19]. Although from reports the incidence of gastric cancer is low in Africa when compared to other regions of the world, this low incidence may be attributed to many factors, such as underreporting (few studies from the region), limited diagnostic facilities (CT scan and endoscopy machines) as well as poor data gathering and keeping. Most reports take into account data obtained from cancer registries that are based only in tertiary health centres located only in urban areas, whose data is mainly from endoscopic biopsies and surgically resected specimens. The majority of the patients in Africa are in the rural areas, mostly attended to by primary care physicians in general hospitals and private clinics where there are neither endoscopic facilities nor histopathologists for histologic diagnosis.

In these centres surgically resected specimens are discarded due to a lack of histopathologists, as such majority of specimens from these peripheral hospitals do not actually reach the cancer registries, thus depriving them of this vital data. Secondly, many patients die before endoscopic or radiologic confirmation of the diagnosis or surgical intervention due to late presentation having wasted valuable time consulting herbal medicine men, and autopsy is not accepted because of religious and cultural taboo. In addition, there is a paucity of data in Africa on genetic factors in gastric cancer patients, therefore it is not fully known whether genetics contribute to the low incidence of gastric cancer reported in the literature as discussions are mainly centred only around modifiable risk factors.

Mortality from gastric cancer continues to be high, with less than 20% of gastric cancer diagnosed in early stages in the US and Europe and 5-year survival rates around 30%. The overall unfavorable prognosis is mainly related to an advanced stage of the disease at the time of presentation to physicians. This may be attributed to treatment guidelines discouraging endoscopic screening of young persons and those without overt alarm features. In Japan and Korea, endoscopy-based mass screening programmes have led to the diagnosis of gastric cancer in the early stages and the 5-year survival rates have increased well above 60% [20–22]. Likewise in Korea, early detection of gastric cancer through national and public screening programmes and advancements in treatment resulted in the proportion of surgically treated early gastric cancer increasing from 28.6 to 63.6%, and the 5-year survival increased from 43.9 to 77.5% [23, 24]. It should be noted that early gastric cancer has an excellent prognosis with a 5-year survival rate of >90% and can often be treated with minimally invasive, organ-sparing modalities, such as endoscopic resection (**Table 1**) [25].

	Incidence				Mortality rate			
	< 60 years		≥ 60 years		< 60 years		≥ 60 years	
World region	**# of cases**	**% of all cases**	**# of cases**	**% of all cases**	**# of cases**	**% of all cases**	**# of cases**	**% of all cases**
1. Africa	2822	42.5	3659	57.6	2284	39.8	3305	60.2
(East-Africa)	4647	46.7	5314	53.3	3824	43.9	4891	56.1
2. America	6316	22.6	14,105	71.7	4168	25.1	12,527	74.9
(South-America)	13,728	27.7	35,819	72.3	9745	24.9	29,420	75.1
3. Asia	58,639	35.1	121,480	65.0	36,646	31.3	107,156	68.7
(Eastern Asia)	170,428	26.0	485,921	74.0	95,223	21.9	339,988	79.1
4. Europe	6692	18.4	27,318	81.6	4115	15.3	20,134	84.7
(Central-eastern Europe)	14,425	22.0	51,091	78.0	9948	19.9	40,070	80.1
5. Oceania	266	29.4	844	70.6	126	24.0	495	76.1
(Australia/New Zealand)	570	21.3	2106	78.7	228	16.8	1127	83.2

 # = number. Bracket – Highest incidence areas.

Table 1.
Average new cases and mortality rates of gastric cancer by world region and age group (Globocan 2020).

2. Risk factors

Risk factors are different for cardia type and non-cardia type gastric cancer, with gastroesophageal reflux disease (GERD) being the main risk factor for cardia-type gastric cancer, while dietary factors, *H. pylori* infection and low socio-economic factor which lead to poor food preservation techniques like salting, or smoking of meat and fish, as well as prickling of vegetables are all risk factors for the non-cardia gastric cancer.

Several risk factors play an important role in the carcinogenesis of gastric cancer which are broadly grouped into; non-modifiable; (genetic composition of an individual, hormonal factors like estrogen), and modifiable risk factors; (*Helicobacter pylori* infection, high intake of salt, red meat, fat, and smoked fish/meat, and low intake of vegetables and fruits).

Excessive salt intake and dietary consumption of smoked meat or fish as well as consumption of pickled vegetables and saturated fats are associated with an increased risk of gastric cancer. However, a diet high in whole-grain cereals, carotenoids, as well as diet containing fruits, vegetables, and other foods of plant origin that are rich in vitamin C are associated with a reduced risk of gastric cancer.

2.1 Modifiable risk factors

2.1.1 Helicobacter pylori

Helicobacter is a genus of gram-negative, microaerophilic bacteria, which is believed to infect two-thirds of the world population. There is a low prevalence of this infection in developed countries such as Europe UK, and the USA where the prevalence ranges from 30–40% [26]. Transmission can occur by aetrogenic, fecal-oral, and oral-oral routes. *H. pylori* is able to colonize and persist within the gastric lumen and once acquired, it persists, usually for life unless eradicated by antimicrobial therapy. Since the report of Barry Marshall and Robin Warren in 1982 implicating *H. pylori* in gastritis, the bacteria have been implicated as the aetiologic factor in the development of gastric cancer. It was also estimated that *H. pylori* colonization increases the risk of gastric cancer approximately 10-fold, therefore *H. pylori* was subsequently designated as a class 1 carcinogen by the WHO [27]. In developing countries of Asia and Africa, 70–90% of the population is infected with *H. pylori*, acquired mostly before the age of 10 years [5, 28, 29]. Similarly, reports from developed countries also suggest that most infections are acquired in childhood.

There is a high prevalence of *H. pylori* in resource-poor regions of the world, particularly in Africa, and Asia which have the highest burden of the infection. Unfortunately, resistance to some of the antibiotics used (**Table 1**) in its treatment is posing a huge challenge in eradicating the pathogen, leading to a high recurrence of dyspeptic symptoms, and the development of gastric adenocarcinoma even in patients who have completed *H. pylori* eradication therapy in these regions.

H. pylori is the common environmental risk factor for atrophic gastritis and gastric cancer. It is likely that atrophic gastritis and intestinal metaplasia represent intermediary steps to gastric cancer. Studies from *Helicobacter pylori* endemic areas showed that atrophic gastritis with or without intestinal metaplasia, was associated with gastric cancer. Similarly, the achlorhydria associated with *H. pylori*-induced gastritis favors the growth of bacteria capable of converting nitrates to nitrites. It was also found that the nitrosamine *N*-methyl-N′-nitro-*N*-nitrosoguanidine causes a high rate of induction

Continent	Antibiotic profile				
	Amo	Metro	Tet	Cla	Lev
Africa	40.8–90.8%	75–100%	50–100%	0–5.5%	0–15%
Asia	23.6%	46.6%	7.4%	27.5%	25.3%
South America	6.6%	53.0%	0	12.9%	21.2%
North America	2.0%	30.5%	0	30.8%	19.0%
Europe	0.4%	31.2%	1.2%	22.1%	14.2%

Amo = Amoxicillin, Metro = Metronidazole; Tet = Tetracycline; Cla = Clarithromycin; Lev = Levofloxacin.

Table 2.
Helicobacter pylori *antibiotic resistance in some continents.*

of adenocarcinoma in the glandular stomach of rats. It should be noted however, that most patients with atrophic gastritis do not develop gastric cancer, suggesting that neither atrophic gastritis nor achlorhydria is solely responsible for the development of gastric cancer, genetic as well as other dietary factors confer additional synergy as pro-carcinogens. Nitrates present in many foods appear to be additional dietary constituents that may act as pro-carcinogens in the GI tract. Nitrates from diet can be converted by bacterial action in a hypochlorhydric stomach to nitrites and subsequently to mutagenic nitrosamines [30]. These events may explain the correlation between dietary intake of foods high in nitrates and the incidence of gastric cancer in different populations (**Table 2**).

2.1.1.1 Amoxicillin

A study by Bello et al. revealed *H. pylori* antimicrobial resistance rate of 90.8% for amoxicillin [31], while Jaka et al. in a systematic review and meta-analysis involving 26 articles reported a 72.6% *H. pylori* resistance to amoxicillin [32] and concluded that prevalence of amoxicillin, metronidazole, and clarithromycin resistance is high in the developing world, which could impair the first-line triple therapy of *H. pylori* infection. A study in China [33] reported a rate of 28.1%, while studies from Malaysia, Saudi Arabia, and Lebanon reported 100, 99, and 100% sensitivity to amoxicillin, respectively [34–37] These differences in antibiotic susceptibility could be attributed to the differences in local antibiotic prescription practice in the various countries at the time of the studies. Studies have shown that in Africa amoxicillin and ampicillin are the most abused antibiotics in both rural and urban areas because they are cheaply available in oral formulations off the counter (**Figures 1** and **2**) [38].

2.1.1.2 Clarithromycin

In a meta-analysis of 178 studies, Alessia et al. showed that clarithromycin resistance was ≥15% in 11 of 15 countries, with the highest rates in Israel (47%; 95% CI, 39–56) and France (43%; 95% CI, 28–57) [39]. In Southeast Asia Region, clarithromycin resistance was significantly increased from 13% (95% CI, 4–22%) in 2006–2008 to 21% (95% CI, 1–42%) in 2012–2016 ($P < .001$), crossing the intervention threshold in 10 years [40]. Clarithromycin resistance the world over was reported as low, ranging from 0–45% [36, 37, 41]. Studies from Malaysia [35] reported 97.9% and in the United States 93.9% sensitivity [39, 42, 43]. In Nigeria, *H. pylori* sensitivity to clarithromycin

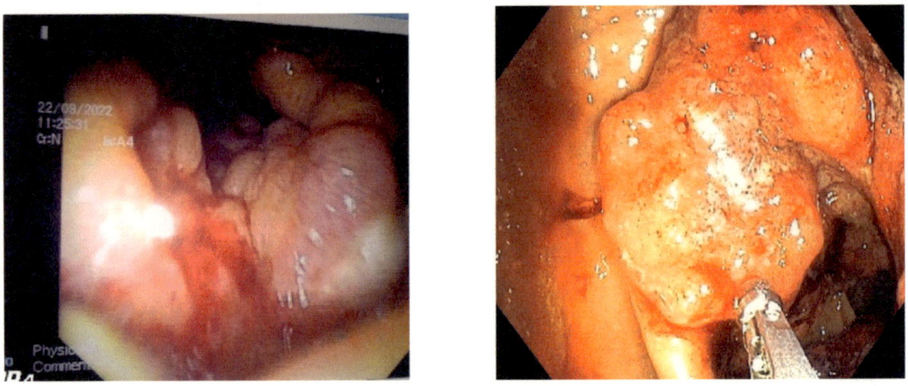

Figure 1.
Endoscopic image of gastric cancer.

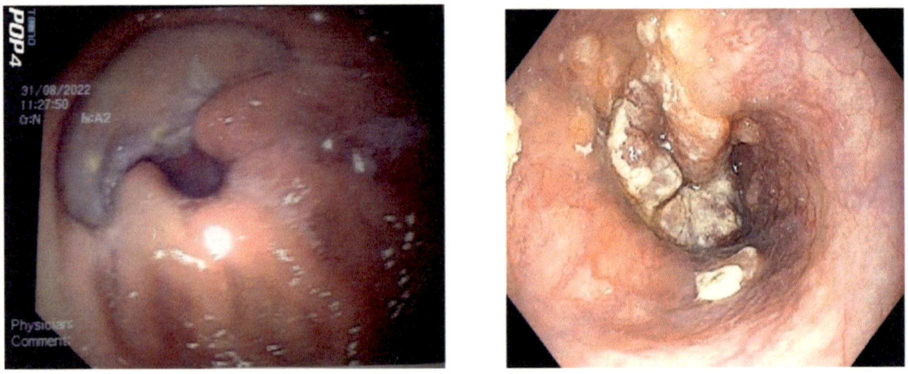

Figure 2.
Histology and CT scan confirmed malignant gastric ulcer.

was 100% [31], which was similar to the study by Kimanga et al. in Kenya [40], Rizwan et al. in Saudi [36], and Sharara et al. in Beirut [37] who reported 100, 96, and 96% clarithromycin susceptibility, respectively. However, Kumala et al. in Indonesia [44] and a study from Cameroon [34] reported lower rates of clarithromycin susceptibility of 72.2 and 55.3% respectively.

2.1.1.3 Metronidazole

Studies in Cameroon, Indonesia, and China reported 93.2, 63.9, and 100% resistance to metronidazole, respectively [34, 39, 45] Metronidazole resistance has been reported in 10–50% of patients in developed countries, [46] whereas in developing countries virtually all strains of *H. pylori* have been found to be resistant to metronidazole [47, 48]. A high resistance rate of 100% observed for metronidazole was observed in Nigeria [31] which is similar to numerous studies from many developing countries that have reported similar results. Metronidazole resistance is the most prevalent pattern of resistance worldwide. Both primary and secondary resistance are well above the threshold, with the highest level recorded in the eastern areas of the world (Eastern Mediterranean Region 56 and 65%, Southeast Asia Region 51 and

44%, and Western Pacific Region 47 and 62%) [38]. Metronidazole resistance had been detected at rates >15% in all the continents (America 44%, Africa 92%, Asia 37%, and Europe 17%) [38]. The highest rates were recorded in Malaysia (82%; 95% CI, 75%—88%) and in China (77%; 95% CI, 74%—79%) [38].

2.1.1.4 Tetracycline

Studies in China and Malaysia [33, 35] reported *H. pylori* resistance rates of 1.2 and 0% respectively to tetracycline, and Sharara in Beirut [37] also reported 2% tetracycline resistance. In Nigeria, there was 100% *H. pylori* resistance to tetracycline [33, 35]. Tetracycline is not currently used for *H. pylori* eradication in Africa because of its high resistance profile.

2.1.1.5 Levofloxacin

Levofloxacin resistance was ≥15% in 5 of 15 countries: 30% (95% CI, 21%—39%) in Turkey, 29% (95% CI, 18%—41%) in Belgium, 18% (95% CI, 15%—22%) in Germany, 16% (95% CI, 14%—18%) in Spain, and 15% (95% CI, 12%—18%) in France [38]. In Nigeria, levofloxacin sensitivity was 100% [31], also in Malaysia, Norazah et al. [35] reported 99% sensitivity to levofloxacin, while a systemic review [47] showed a susceptibility rate of 88.4% in Asia, 75.9% in Europe. Levofloxacin resistance in Western Pacific Region in a study by Alessia et al. [38] showed a significant increase from 12% (95% CI, 8%—17%) in 2006—2008 to 31% (95% CI, 27%—36%) in 2012—2016 ($P < .001$).

Helicobacter pylori a bacterial pathogen was found to be a causative agent of gastric cancer with high prevalence in low-income countries and also in continents with the highest population in the world. Increased resistance to antibiotics used in *H. pylori* infection is posing a major challenge to its eradication. In limited-resource countries, there is poor hygiene and sanitation with poor drinking water that is mostly sourced from wells or flowing streams contaminated with feces as a result of open defaecation. In addition, there are no local *H. pylori* treatment guidelines that consider local antibiotic susceptibility, with none availability and affordability of diagnostics facilities to monitor *H. pylori* eradication. These problems if tackled will mitigate the spread of this bacteria and lead to its eradication.

3. High dietary salt

Salt is an important ingredient that gives food its desired taste and has also been in use for centuries as a food preservative. It is the excess intake of salt in diet, and not salt per se, that is positively associated with the risk of gastric cancer. Excess salt in diet has long been thought to be an aetiological agent of stomach cancer, but not until 1959 when it was first reported as a possible risk factor for stomach cancer. A meta-analysis by Sheng Ge et al. showed that high salt intake was significantly associated with a 105% greater risk of gastric cancer compared with low salt intake (OR = 2.05 95% CI [1.60, 2.62]; = 154.7; $P < 0.00001$) [49–51].

Several epidemiological studies have investigated the association between salted foods and risk of gastric cancer. In 2005 a study estimated the average daily salt intake in the Korean population and was found to be 13.4 g, which was far beyond 5 g daily salt intake recommended by the World Health Organization [52–54]. Furthermore, poor socio-economic status was found to be associated with the use of pickled vegetables and also with a high prevalence of *H. pylori* infection. Traditional processing of pickling vegetables in some regions of China, Japan, and Korea involves the fermentation of local vegetables, with or without adding salt. This processing and the high salt intake are associated with the formation of N-nitrosamines, which were found to be carcinogenic [55]. Studies of high-risk populations showed that genotoxic agents such as *N*-nitroso compounds formed in the human stomach from ingested nitrates in the diet may play a role in pathogenesis of gastric tumor. High mortality rates from gastric cancer were also noted in areas with high nitrate concentrations in soil and drinking water.

Ingestion of salt directly damages the stomach lining, enhancing the carcinogenic effects of gastric carcinogens, increasing nitroso compound formation, and facilitating *H. pylori* infection [52]. Mucosal cell proliferation in the antrum of the stomach was positively correlated with salt intake in *H. pylori*-positive patients, but no relationship was found in patients without *H. pylori* [52]. An endoscopy-based Asian study confirmed that high salt intake could be associated with an increased risk of atrophic gastritis and with intestinal metaplasia, dysplasia, and carcinoma [56]. Similarly, a European study concluded that an increased risk of gastric dysplasia or gastric cancer in patients with *H. pylori* infection is further enhanced by high salt intake [57]. A Korean case–control study investigating the role of salt and *H. pylori* infection in stomach cancer found that subjects with *H. pylori* infection and high salt consumption had a 10-fold risk of early stomach cancer compared with subjects with low salt consumption but without *H. pylori* infection ($P = 0.047$) [58]. Similarly, another study conducted in Japan evaluated the potential interaction between diet and *H. pylori*, and found a positive association between increased salt intake and gastric cancer that was statistically significant only among subjects with *H. pylori* infection [59]. High dietary salt intake may potentiate the colonization of *H. pylori*, a known risk factor for gastric cancer, through the increase of surface mucous cell mucin and decrease of gland mucous cell mucin [57]. High salt intake causes damage to the gastric epithelium and provokes inflammatory responses which may increase epithelial cell proliferation as part of the repair process and increase the probability of endogenous mutations [51, 60]. Another mechanism of high salt action in gastric carcinogenesis is the induction of hypergastrinemia. Gastrin itself may mediate epithelial cell growth in *H. pylori*-colonized mucosa and chronic hypergastrinemia can synergize with *H. pylori* infection leading to parietal cell loss and progression to gastric cancer. Furthermore, poor socio-economic status was found to be associated with the use of pickled vegetables and also with a high prevalence of *H. pylori* infection [50].

Long-term use of a refrigerator has been suggested to decrease stomach cancer risk [61]. Even though, there is no direct relation between refrigerators with gastric cancer, but refrigerator use may cause a change in dietary habits that discourages the consumption of salted and smoked meat or fish, as well as increasing the storage and consumption of fresh fruit and vegetables. In low-income countries such as Asia and Africa, refrigerators are still not much in use despite their advent almost two centuries ago. Refrigerators are still not affordable, and even when available, there is a scarcity of electricity to power the appliance. These problems have led to the retention of the old practice of preserving foods by pickling, salting, curing, and smoking. Therefore, preserved foods in general may be eaten more by those to whom refrigeration is not available.

4. Smoked fish and meat

Meat and fish preserved by smoking, curing, and pickling contain high levels of nitrosamines, nitro compounds, polycyclic aromatic hydrocarbons (in smoked meats), or heterocyclic amines [62] which have been found to be both mutagens and carcinogens and have thus been classified as carcinogenic to humans. People who consumed smoked-dried salted beef on a regular basis had a nearly three-fold increased risk of gastric cancer [63]. Among processed foods, smoked foods seem to be involved in gastric carcinogenesis through the formation of polycyclic aromatic hydrocarbon [2]. Much evidence indicates that cooking conditions and dietary habits can contribute to human cancer risk through the ingestion of gene-toxic compounds from heat-processed foods. The genotoxic and carcinogenic potential of these cooked foods have been evaluated regularly by the International Agency for Research on Cancer (IARC), which has come to the conclusion that several of these food-borne toxicants found in cooked foods are possibly carcinogenic to humans [55]. It has been found that the consumption of charcoal-grilled beef or broiled meat and fish was associated with an increased risk of gastric cancer, but total meat consumption was not associated with gastric cancer risk in case-control studies [52, 64]. A study in Mali found that 57.5% of their patients with gastric cancer regularly consume fish preserved by salting and smoking. Similar findings were reported by authors from other African sub-regions where over 80% of gastric cancer patients consume salted foods with potash cereal dough [30].

5. Fat

An inverse association was observed in a meta-analysis between vegetable fat intake and gastric cancer risk but found no association with animal fat. Results from this meta-analysis indicate a possible significant positive association between saturated fat, as well as total fat intake and gastric cancer risk [65, 66]. Even though the mechanisms by which fat increases the risk of gastric cancer are still not established, high cholesterol intake causes impairments in apo-lipoproteins and lipids, which may lead to inflammation. High-fat diets have been found to increase the risk of gastric cancer due to their obesogenic effects and the resulting inflammatory response. Findings revealed that intakes of fat (total, saturated, unsaturated, omega-6 fatty acids, and cholesterol) were significantly associated with gastric cancer. In Canada and the US, a study on the relationship between dietary habits and the development of gastric cancer found that a Western diet which mostly contains processed meats, refined grains, fats, and sugars, was associated with an 86% increased risk of developing gastric cancer among women and a 44% increased risk among men. However, the diet that included increased consumption of fruits, vegetables, and fish was associated with a 60% decreased risk of developing gastric cancer among women and a 54% decreased risk among men. This finding, like others, provides proof that dietary habits significantly reduce the risk of developing cancers [67].

6. Protective factors of gastric cancer

6.1 Whole grain

Xiao-Feng et al. in a systematic review and meta-analysis first reported the association between whole grains and digestive tract cancer, and the result shows that higher intake of whole grains can reduce the risk of gastric cancer, oesophageal cancer, and colorectal cancer. Several studies have found a lower risk of gastric cancer associated with a higher intake of whole grains which can occur through a variety of mechanisms [68–71]. Whole grains are an important source of dietary fiber which can increase fecal load and thus shorten the transit time through the intestines, thus reducing the contact time between carcinogens and the intestinal epithelium. Dietary fiber is also fermented in the colon into short-chain fatty acids which have the potential to promote apoptosis and anti-tumour activity, thereby reducing tumor growth. Additionally, it was reported that dietary fiber can remove nitrite in the stomach and reduce the concentration of nitroso compounds [72–75]. Reports also found that whole grains have antioxidant and anti-inflammatory properties and can improve blood sugar response and reduce insulin resistance, thereby reducing the risk of cancer [75]. In general, intake of whole grain was associated with significantly lower cancer risk [76], and these findings are consistent with reports and recommendations that advocate for a higher consumption of whole grains [76]. In resource-limited countries of Africa, foods mainly are of whole grains with lots of vegetables and fruits that are sourced from farms. This protective dietary habit, in spite of the high *H. pylori* incidence, may be a factor contributing to the low incidence of gastric cancer in Africa which could further shed more light on the suggested "African-enigma" in gastric cancer.

6.2 Fresh fruits and vegetables

Many studies have shown the benefit of fruit and vegetable intake in lowering gastric cancer risk. A large multicentric prospective study from Japan with a 10-year follow-up of 40,000 patients reported an inverse correlation between gastric cancer with the intake of fruit and vegetables [77]. A meta-analysis of cohort studies also confirmed an inverse association between fruit and vegetable intake and gastric cancer [78]. The beneficial effect of fruit and vegetable intake could be due to the presence of high levels of vitamins, ascorbic acid, carotenoid, and catechins which have antioxidant effects and anticancer activities thus reducing the risk of developing gastric cancer [2]. Two independent systematic review and meta-analysis found that a 100 g/day increase in fruit consumption was statistically significant and leads to reduced gastric cancer risk by 5 and 40% respectively [14, 79, 80]. Another meta-analysis also found an inverse relationship between intake of citrus fruit and risk of cardia-type gastric cancer and noted that vitamin C-containing fruits trap oxygen free-radicals, preventing DNA oxidation through the provision of antioxidant effects and thus regulating cell proliferation and apoptosis [14, 81]. Fruits decrease DNA damage by directly inhibiting the expression of CYP1A1; a cytochrome P450 enzyme that metabolizes toxins into carcinogens. The phytochemical antioxidants in fruit could also reduce free-radical damage caused by *H. pylori*-induced inflammation.

7. Conclusion

Gastric cancer is declining in Europe and America, but in Asia, Middle East, and Africa which have high incidences of *H. pylori*, the disease is yet to receive government attention because emphasis is still being placed on communicable diseases allowing gastric cancer to become a major threat to young adults and the elderly.

In resource-limited countries, dietary protective factors against gastric cancer are firmly in place and only need to be emphasized. In rural and semi-urban areas, *H. pylori* infection is widespread, but the food is made from whole grains, with abundant fresh fruits and vegetables readily available because they are sourced from nearby farms and gardens. While in cities, there is low *H. pylori* infection, however, there are abundant restaurants that serve fast foods made of processed meats or fish, refined grains, high sugars, and fried and fatty foods with little or no vegetables. Such a diet is only rich in the risk factors and poor in gastric cancer protective factors. Eradicating *H. pylori* requires a holistic approach by governments, and non-governmental organizations in the area of increased budgetary allocation to education and health, provision of portable and clean drinking water, poverty eradication policies, improved sanitation as well as regulation and control of antibiotic use/abuse. Without having these measures in place, eradicating *H. pylori*, and reducing gastric cancer incidence will be difficult if not impossible in low-income regions of the world.

Author details

Ahmad Bello Kumo[1,2]

1 Faculty of Clinical Sciences, Departments of Internal Medicine, Ahmadu Bello, Zaria, Nigeria

2 Ahmadu Bello University Teaching Hospital, Zaria, Nigeria

*Address all correspondence to: akbello06@gmail.com

References

[1] Bray F, Ferlay J, Soerjomataram I, Siegel RL, Torre LA, Jemal A. Global cancer statistics 2018: GLOBOCAN estimates of incidence and mortality worldwide for 36 cancers in 185 countries. CA: A Cancer Journal for Clinicians. 2018;**68**:394-424

[2] Eusebi L, H, Telese A, Marasco G, Bazzoli F, Zagar RM. Gastric cancer prevention strategies: A global perspective. Journal of Gastroenterology and Hepatology. 2020;**35**:1495-1502

[3] Thrift AP, El-Serag HB. Burden of gastric cancer. Clinical Gastroenterology and Hepatology. 2019;**18**:534-542

[4] Sung H, Ferlay J, Siegel RL, Laversanne M, Soerjomataram I, Jemal A, et al. Global cancer statistics 2020: GLOBOCAN estimates of incidence and mortality worldwide for 36 cancers in 185 countries. CA: A Cancer Journal for Clinicians. 2021;**71**:209-249. DOI: 10.3322/caac.21660

[5] Bello AK, Umar AB, Borodo MM. Prevalence and risk factors for *Helicobacter pylori* infection in gastroduodenal diseases in Kano, Nigeria. African Journal of Medical and Health Sciences. 2018;**17**:41-46. DOI: 10.4103/ajmhs.ajmhs_36_17

[6] Janice O, Abboud Y, Burch M, Gong J, Waters K, Ghaith J, et al. Rising incidence of non-cardia gastric cancer among young women in the United States, 2000-2018: A time-trend analysis using the USCS database. Cancers (Basel). 2023;**15**(8):2283. Published online 2023 Apr 13. DOI: 10.3390/cancers15082283

[7] Ajani JA, D'Amico TA, Bentrem DJ, Chao J, Cooke D, Corvera C. NCCN clinical practice guidelines in oncology gastric cancer, version 2.2022. Journal of the National Comprehensive Cancer Network. 2022;**20**(2):167-192. DOI: 10.6004/jnccn.2022.0008

[8] Merchant SJ, Kim J, Choi AH, Sun V, Chao J, Nelson R. A rising trend in the incidence of advanced gastric cancer in young Hispanic men. Gastric Cancer. 2017;**20**(2):226-234

[9] Camargo MC, Anderson WF, King JB, et al. Divergent trends for gastric cancer incidence by anatomical subsite in US adults. Gut. 2011;**60**:1644-1649

[10] Crew KD, Neugut AI. Epidemiology of gastric cancer. World Journal of Gastroenterology. 2006;**12**:354-362

[11] Hu B, El Hajj N, Sittler S, et al. Gastric cancer: Classification, histology and application of molecular pathology. Journal of Gastrointestinal Oncology. 2012;**3**:251-261

[12] Sitarz R, Skierucha M, Mielko J, et al. Gastric cancer: Epidemiology, prevention, classification, and treatment. Cancer Management and Research. 2018;**10**:239-248

[13] National Cancer Institute. Surveillance, epidemiology, and end results (SEER) program. In: Cancer Stat Facts: Stomach Cancer. National Cancer Institute; 2021

[14] Yang W-J, Zhao H-P, Yan Y, Wang J-H, Guo L, Liu J-Y, et al. Updates on global epidemiology, risk and prognostic factors of gastric cancer. World Journal of Gastroenterology. 2023;**29**(16):2452-2468. Published online 2023 Apr 28. DOI: 10.3748/wjg.v29.i16.2452

[15] Thrift AP, El-Serag HB. Burden of gastric cancer. Clinical Gastroenterology and Hepatology. 2020;**18**(3):534-542. Published online 2019Jul27. DOI: 10.1016/j.cgh.2019.07.045

[16] Bashir MT, Adamu AS, Musa MB, Kumo BA. Severe bone pain as first presentation of gastric malignancy. Nigerian Journal of Basic and Clinical Sciences. 2013;**10**(2):91-94

[17] Bang GA, Savom EP, Oumarou BN, Ngamy CKM, Moto GB, et al. Clinical epidemiology and mortality risk factors of gastric cancer in a sub-Saharan African setting: A retrospective analysis of 120 cases in Yaoundé (Cameroon). The Pan African Medical Journal. 2020;**37**:104. Published online 2020 Sep 30. DOI: 10.11604/pamj.2020.37.104.25422

[18] Mellouki I, Iaazar N, Benyachou B, Aqodad N, Ibrahim A. Epidemiologie du cancer gastrique: experience d'un centre hospitalier marocain. Panafrican Medical Journal. 2014;**17**:42

[19] Dembélé BT, Togo A, Kanté L, Traoré A, Diakité I, Tounkara Y, et al. Non-resectable gastric cancers at the Department of General Surgery at CHU Gabriel Touré, Bamako. Le Mali Médical. 2012;**27**(1):14-18

[20] Bagnan KO, Padonou N, Kodjoh N, Houansou T. Le cancer de l'estomac: à propos de 51 cas observés au CNHU de Cotonou. Médecine d'Afrique Noire. 1994;**41**(1):39-43

[21] Huang RJ, Hwang JH. Improving the early diagnosis of gastric cancer. Gastrointestinal Endoscopy Clinics of North America. 2021;**31**(3):503-517. DOI: 10.1016/j.giec.2021.03.005

[22] Lui FH, Tuan B, Swenson SL, et al. Ethnic disparities in gastric cancer incidence and survival in the USA: An updated analysis of 1992-2009 SEER data. Digestive Diseases and Sciences. 2014;**59**:3027-3034

[23] Kim T-H, Kim I-H, Kang SJ, Choi M, Kim B-H, Eom BW, et al. Korean practice guidelines for gastric cancer 2022: An evidence-based, multidisciplinary approach. Journal of Gastric Cancer. 2023;**23**(1):3-106. Published online 2023 Jan 31. DOI: 10.5230/jgc.2023.23.e11

[24] Information Committee of the Korean Gastric Cancer Association. Korean gastric cancer association-led nationwide survey on surgically treated gastric cancers in 2019. Journal of Gastric Cancer. 2021;**21**:221-235

[25] Suzuki H, Oda I, Abe S, Sekiguchi M, Mori G, Nonaka S, et al. High rate of 5-year survival among patients with early gastric cancer undergoing curative endoscopic submucosal dissection. Gastric Cancer. 2016;**19**:198-205. DOI: 10.1007/s10120-015-0469-0

[26] Saad RJ, Chey WD. Persistent *Helicobacter pylori* infection after a course of antimicrobial therapy – What's next? Clinical Gastroenterology and Hepatology. 2008;**6**:1086-1090

[27] Anwar BK, Armstrong P, Correa D, Forman JM, Gentile M, Haswell-Elkins, et al. Schistosomes, liver flukes and *Helicobacter pylori*. IARC Monographs on the Evaluation of Carcinogenic Risks to Human. 1994;**61**:3-12

[28] Salih BA. *Helicobacter pylori* infection in developing countries: The burden for how long? Saudi Journal of Gastroenterology. 2009;**15**(3):201-207

[29] Asrat D, Nilsson I, Mengistu Y, et al. Prevalence of *Helicobacter pylori*

infection among adult dyspeptic patients in Ethiopia. Annals of Tropical Medicine & Parasitology. 2004;**98**(2):181-189

[30] Sanogo S, Traoré D, Coulibaly M, Togola B, Bengaly B, Touré OI, et al. Environmental risk factors for stomach cancer in an African setting about 193 cases at the CHU point G in Bamako/ Mali. Surgical Science. 2021;**12**:23-30. DOI: 10.4236/ss.2021.122004

[31] Bello AK, Borodo MM, Yakasai AM, Tukur AD. *Helicobacter pylori* antibiotic sensitivity pattern in dyspeptic patients in Kano, Nigeria. Southern African Journal of Infectious Diseases. 2019;**34**(1):a125. DOI: 10.4102/sajid.v34i1.125

[32] Jaka H, Rhee JA, Ostlundh L, et al. The magnitude of antibiotic resistance to *Helicobacter pylori* in Africa and identified mutations which confer resistance to antibiotics: Systematic review and meta-analysis. BMC Infectious Diseases. 2018;**18**(1):193. DOI: 10.1186/s12879-018-3099-4

[33] Wu H, Shi XD, Wang HT, Liu JX. Resistance of *Helicobacter pylori* to metronidazole, tetracycline and amoxycillin. Journal of Antimicrobial Chemotherapy. 2000;**46**(1):121-123. DOI: 10.1093/jac/46.1.121

[34] Roland NN, Alertia EMT, Juliet EAO, et al. *Helicobacter pylori* isolates recovered from gastric biopsies of patients with gastro-duodenal pathologies in Cameroon: Current status of antibiogram. Tropical Medicine & International Health. 2008;**13**(6):848-854

[35] Norazah A, Zakaria WR, Mohamed R. Analysis of antibiotic susceptibility patterns of *Helicobacter pylori* isolates from Malaysia. Helicobacter. 2010;**16**(1):47-51. DOI: 10.1111/j.1523-5378.2010.00816.x

[36] Rizwan M, Fatima N, Ayesha A. Epidemiology and pattern of antibiotic resistance in *Helicobacter pylori*: Scenario from Saudi Arabia. Saudi Journal of Gastroenterology. 2014;**20**(4):212-218. DOI: 10.4103/1319-3767.136935

[37] Sharara A, Marwan C, George FA, Kassem AB, Fadi HM. Prevalence of *Helicobacter pylori* resistance to metronidazole, clarithromycin, amoxycillin and tetracycline in Lebanon. International Journal of Antimicrobial Agents. 2002;**19**(2):155-158. DOI: 10.1016/S0924-8579(01)00482-4

[38] Gebeyetu E, Bantie L, Azage M. Inappropraite use of antibiotics and its associated factors among urban and rural communities of Bahir Dar city administration North-West Ethiopia. PLoS One. 2015;**10**(9):e0138179. DOI: 10.1371/journal.pone.0138179

[39] Savoldi A, Carrara E, Graham DY, Conti M, Tacconelli E. Prevalence of antibiotic resistance in *Helicobacter pylori*: A systematic review and meta-analysis in world health organization regions. Gastroenterology. 2018;**155**(5):1372-1382

[40] Bai P, Zhou LY, Xiao XM, Luo Y, Ding Y. Antibiotic susceptibility profile of *Helicobacter pylori* isolated from Chinese patients. Journal of Digestive Diseases. 2015;**16**(8):2980

[41] Kimang'a AN, Revathi G, Kariuki S, Sayed S, Devani S. *Helicobacter pylori*: Prevalence and antibiotic susceptibility among Kenyans. South African Medical Journal. 2010;**100**(1):53-57

[42] Adamek RJ, Suerbaum S, Pfaffenbach B, Opfenkuch W. Primary acquired *Helicobacter pylori* resistance to clarithromycin, metronidazole and amoxicillin influence on treatment

outcome. The American Journal of Gastroenterology. 1998;**93**(3):386-389. DOI: 10.1111/j.1572-0241.1998.00386.x

[43] Everhart JE, Kruszon-Moran D, Perez-Perez GI, Tralka TS, McQuillan G. Seroprevalence and ethnic differences in *Helicobacter pylori* infection among adults in the United States. The Journal of Infectious Diseases. 2000;**181**(4):1359-1363. DOI: 10.1086/315384

[44] Kumala W, Aziz R. Patterns of *Helicobacter pylori* isolate resistance to fluoroquinolones, amoxicillin, and metronidazoles. The Southeast Asian Journal of Tropical Medicine and Public Health. 2006;**37**(5):1260

[45] De Francesco V, Giorgio F, Hassan C, et al. Worldwide *H. pylori* antibiotic resistance: A systematic review. Journal of Gastrointestinal and Liver Diseases. 2010;**19**(4):409-414

[46] Nahar S, Mukhopadhyay AK, Khan R, et al. Antimicrobial susceptibility of *Helicobacter pylori* strains isolated in Bangladesh. Journal of Clinical Microbiology. 2004;**42**(10):4856-4858. DOI: 10.1128/JCM.42.10.4856-4858.2004

[47] Goodwin A, Kersulyte D, Sisson G, Veldhuyzen van Zanten SJ, Berg DE, Hoffman PS. Metronidazole resistance in *Helicobacter pylori* is due to null mutations in a gene (rdxA) that encodes an oxygen-insensitive NADPH nitroreductase. Molecular Microbiology. 1998;**28**(2):383-393. DOI: 10.1046/j.1365-2958.1998.00806.x

[48] Oladiipo AA, Abdul RA, Babatunde WO, et al. Antibiotic resitance of *Helicobacter pylori* from patients in Ille-Ife, south-west, Nigeria. African Health Sciences. 2007;**7**(3):143-147

[49] Sato T, Fukuyama T, Suzuki T, Takayanagi J, Murakami T, Shiotsuki N, et al. Studies of causation of gastric cancer 2. The relation between gastric cancer mortality rate and salted food intake in several places in Japan. Bulletin of National Institute of Health Sciences. 1959;**8**:187-198

[50] Wang X-Q, Terry PD, Yan H. Review of salt consumption and stomach cancer risk: Epidemiological and biological evidence. World Journal of Gastroenterology. 2009;**15**(18):2204-2213. Published online 2009 May 14. DOI: 10.3748/wjg.15.2204

[51] Ge S, Feng X, Shen L, Wei Z, Zhu Q, Sun J. Association between habitual dietary salt intake and risk of gastric cancer: A systematic review of observational studies. Gastroenterology Research and Practice. 2012;**2012**:808120, 11 pages. DOI: 10.1155/2012/808120

[52] Shin A, Kim J, Park S. Gastric cancer epidemiology in Korea. Journal of Gastric Cancer. 2011;**11**(3):135-140. Published online 2011 Sep 29. DOI: 10.5230/jgc.2011.11.3.135

[53] World Health Organization. Salt Reduction. World Health Organization; 2023. ISBN 9789240069985

[54] Hyseni L, Elliot-Green A, Lloyd-Williams F, Kypridemos C, O'Flaherty M, McGill R, et al. Systematic review of dietary salt reduction policies: Evidence for an effectiveness hierarchy? PLoS One. 2017;**12**(5):e0177535. Published online 2017 May 18. DOI: 10.1371/journal.pone.0177535

[55] Jagerstad M, Skog K. Genotoxicity of heat-processed foods. Mutation Research. 2005;**574**:156-172

[56] Song JH, Kim YS, Heo NJ, Lim JH, Yang SY, Chung GE, et al. High salt

intake is associated with atrophic gastritis with intestinal metaplasia. Cancer Epidemiology, Biomarkers & Prevention. 2017;**26**(7):1133-1138

[57] Gaddy JA, Radin JN, Loh JT, Feng Zhang MK, Washington RM, Peek Jr et al. High dietary salt intake exacerbates Helicobacter pylori-induced gastric carcinogenesis. Infection and Immunity. 2013;**81**(6):2258-2267. DOI: 10.1128/IAI.01271-12

[58] Rocco A, Nardone G. Diet, *H pylori* infection and gastric cancer: Evidence and controversies. World Journal of Gastroenterology. 2007;**13**(21):2901-2912. Published online 2007 Jun 7. DOI: 10.3748/wjg.v13.i21.2901

[59] Tsugane S, Sasazuki S, Kobayashi M, Sasaki S. Salt and salted food intake and subsequent risk of gastric cancer among middle-aged Japanese men and women. British Journal of Cancer. 2004;**90**(1):128-134. Published online 2004 Jan 6. DOI: 10.1038/sj.bjc.6601511

[60] Fox JG, Dangler CA, Taylor NS, King A, Koh TJ, Wang TC. High-salt diet induces gastric epithelial hyperplasia and parietal cell loss, and enhances *Helicobacter pylori* colonization in C57BL/6 mice. Cancer Research. 1999;**59**(19):4823-4828

[61] Yan S, Gan Y, Song X, Chen Y, Liao N, Chen S, et al. Association between refrigerator use and the risk of gastric cancer: A systematic review and meta-analysis of observational studies. PLoS One. 2018;**13**(8):e0203120. Published online 2018 Aug 30. DOI: 10.1371/journal.pone.0203120

[62] Afé OHI, Kpoclou YE, Douny C, Anihouvi VB, Igout A, Mahillon J, et al. Chemical hazards in smoked meat and fish. Food Science & Nutrition. 2021;**9**(12):6903-6922. Published online 2021 Oct 18. DOI: 10.1002/fsn3.2633

[63] Richa NS, Sageena G. Dietary factors associated with gastric cancer - a review. Translational Medicine Communications. 2022;**7**:7. DOI: 10.1186/s41231-022-00111-x

[64] Collatuzzo G, Etemadi A, Sotoudeh M, Nikmanesh A, Poustchi H, Khoshnia M, et al. Meat consumption and risk of esophageal and gastric cancer in the Golestan cohort study, Iran. International Journal of Cancer. 2022;**151**:1005-1012

[65] Han J, Jiang Y, Liu X, Meng Q, Xi Q, Zhuang Q, et al. Dietary fat intake and risk of gastric cancer: A meta-analysis of observational studies. PLoS One. 2015;**10**(9):e0138580. DOI: 10.1371/journal.pone.0138580

[66] Allehdan S, Bassil M, Alatrash RM, Al-Jaberi T, Hushki A, Rayyan Y, et al. Macronutrients intake and risk of stomach cancer: Findings from case-control study. Nutrients. 2022;**14**:2373. DOI: 10.3390/nu14122373

[67] Campbell P, Sloan M, Kreiger N. Dietary patterns and risk of incident gastric adenocarcinoma. American Journal of Epidemiology. 2008;**167**:295-304

[68] Yujie X, Yang J, Liang D, Li K, Zhou Y. Association of whole grain, refined grain, and cereal consumption with gastric cancer risk: A meta-analysis of observational studies. Food Science & Nutrition. 2019;7:256-265

[69] Wang T, Zhan R, Lu J, Lu Z, Peng XJ, Wang M. Grain consumption and risk of gastric cancer: A meta-analysis. International Journal of Food Sciences and Nutrition. 2020;**71**(2):164-175. DOI: 10.1080/09637486.2019.1631264

[70] Zhang X-F, Wang X-K, Tang Y-J, Guan X-X, Guo Y, Fan J-M, et al. Association of whole grains intake and the risk of digestive tract cancer: A systematic review and meta-analysis. Nutrition Journal. 2020;**19**:52. Published online 2020 Jun 3. DOI: 10.1186/s12937-020-00556-6), 10.1186/s12937-020-00556-6)

[71] Oh H, Kim H, Lee DH, Lee A, Giovannucci EL, Kang SS, et al. Different dietary fibre sources and risks of colorectal cancer and adenoma: A dose-response meta-analysis of prospective studies. The British Journal of Nutrition. 2019;**122**:605-615

[72] Idehen E, Tang Y, Sang SM. Bioactive phytochemicals in barley. Journal of Food and Drug Analysis. 2017;**25**:148-161

[73] Wiseman M. The second World Cancer Research Fund/American Institute for Cancer Research expert report. Food, nutrition, physical activity, and the prevention of cancer: A global perspective. The Proceedings of the Nutrition Society. 2008;**67**:253-256

[74] McNabney SM, Henagan TM. Short chain fatty acids in the colon and peripheral tissues: A focus on butyrate, colon cancer, obesity and insulin resistance. Nutrients. 2017;**9**:1348. DOI: 10.3390/nu9121348

[75] Călinoiu LF, Vodnar DC. Whole grains and phenolic acids: A review on bioactivity, functionality, health benefits and bioavailability. Nutrients. 2018;**10**:1615. DOI: 10.3390/nu10111615

[76] Gaesser GA. Whole grains, refined grains, and cancer risk: A systematic review of meta-analyses of observational studies. Nutrients. 2020;**12**(12):3756. Published online 2020 Dec 7. DOI: 10.3390/nu12123756

[77] Kobayashi M, Tsubono Y, Sasazuki S, Sasaki S, Tsugane S. Vegetables, fruit and risk of gastric cancer in Japan: A 10-year follow-up of the JPHC study cohort I. International Journal of Cancer. 2002;**102**(1):39-44. DOI: 10.1002/ijc.10659

[78] Naemi Kermanshahi M, Safaei E, Tutunchi H, Naghshi S, Mobarak S, Asadi M, et al. Fruit and vegetable intake in relation to gastric cancer risk: A comprehensive and updated systematic review and dose-response meta-analysis of cohort studies. Frontiers in Nutrition. 2023;**10**:973171. DOI: 10.3389/fnut.2023.973171

[79] Wang Q, Chen Y, Wang X, Gong G, Li G, Li C. Consumption of fruit, but not vegetables, may reduce risk of gastric cancer: Results from a meta-analysis of cohort studies. European Journal of Cancer. 2014;**50**(8):1498-1509

[80] Liao Y-P, Zheng Q-X, Jiang X-M, Chen X-Q, Gao X-X, Pan Y-Q. Fruit, vegetable, and fruit juice consumption and risk of gestational diabetes mellitus: A systematic review and meta-analysis. Liao et al. Nutrition Journal. 2023;**22**:27. DOI: 10.1186/s12937-023-00855-8

[81] Update: As part of the WCRF/AICR. Diet, Nutrition, Physical Activity and Cancer: A Global Perspective Report. Update: As part of the WCRF/AICR; 2018

Chapter 3

Atmospheric Pollution and Toxicological Aspects of *Helicobacter pylori* Infection: Background, Pathophysiology and New Innovative Hypotheses

Josaphat Ndelo di Phanzu, Lievins-Corneille Mputu Malolo, Patrick Ndelo Matondo and Yannick Belo Nuapia

Abstract

A strange phenomenon characterized by numerous pathologies occurred in DR Congo and in some other countries of Subsaharian Africa since a few decades. While the entire population is convinced of massive poisonings provoked by a ritual poison from the eastern Africa, named Karuho, we incredibly established, since 2010, the responsibility of *Helicobacter pylori* in the phenomenon, thanks to cross-sectional epidemiological studies. Our findings have been published in international journals and presented in international scientific forums. The purpose of this chapter is to describe the background and conduct of this research, the pathophysiology of the *Helicobacter pylori* involvement, as well as the new innovative hypotheses on Helicobacter infection generated by this research.

Keywords: *Helicobacter pylori*, toxicological trends, carbon dioxide and ammonia gas, extradigestive pathologies, antiurease, constipation, pathophysiology, innovative hypotheses

1. Introduction

Discovered in 1875 by German researchers and discovered again in 1982 by two Australian researchers, J. Robin Warren and Barry J. Marshall, *Helicobacter pylori* remains in the human stomach, despite the high acidity of this medium. Its discovery in the stomach, along with the announcement of its role in gastritis, gastric ulcer and stomach cancer by J. Robin Warren and Barry J. Marshall, caused great controversy worldwide for more than two decades. Since 2005, when the two Australian researchers won the Nobel Prize, the controversy has stopped as the two researchers' findings have been fully confirmed by other researchers around the world [1–4].

IntechOpen

It is now known that *Helicobacter pylori* tolerates little oxygen, and releases carbon dioxide and ammonia gas into the stomach but is normally unable to cause poisoning because the gases, after their release, become liquid, which prevents them from crossing the digestive barrier. Proton Pump Inhibitors (PPIs) are crucial in the therapy of this infection since the symptoms are primarily digestive [5, 6].

The present research undertaken in the Democratic Republic of Congo since 1990 has established that, contrary to what is reported in the literature, infection with *Helicobacter pylori* can well cause intoxication. Indeed, the carbon dioxide and ammonia it generates in the stomach, can well, under certain circumstances, pass into the blood and produce numerous extradigestive pathologies.

2. Background

2.1 Research design

The research was not designed to study *Helicobacter pylori* infection but to deal with suspicions of massive poisoning that appeared in DR Congo in the early 1980s, almost at the same time as HIV, first in northeastern DR Congo, mainly in Goma and Bukavu, before gradually spreading throughout the country, including the city of Kinshasa. The poison concerned would be a mythical and ritual poison from the east of the country and even from East Africa, extremely virulent, called Karuho poison. Its nature and its symptoms were unknown. Any foreigner traveling to the east of the country, mainly, to Goma and Bukavu, had to develop the unusual symptoms attributed to this unknown mythical poison. The patients were cared for only by traditional healers and self-proclaimed toxicologists, presenting themselves as the only specialists in this poison, since this phenomenon was unknown in the hospital [7–9].

The traditional diagnosis of poisoning, carried out on saliva, is very rudimentary. Early in the morning, the supposedly poisoned person spits into a glass of water after scraping his throat. In the event of a positive test, saliva flows to the bottom of the glass. The treatment is based on honey and various plant extracts, including strong laxatives. The results are more or less good. As the Karuho phenomenon was unknown in hospitals and following the failures of traditional healers' treatments, people suspecting poisoning began to come to the Toxicology Department of the University of Kinshasa to meet the toxicologist. The flow of patients continues until today. The Toxicology Laboratory of the University of Kinshasa is practically the only operational toxicological laboratory in DR Congo, since 1974, although poorly equipped.

Suspicions of poisoning arouse a strong fear of immediate death, everywhere across the country in all walks of life: family, professional, school, academic, political and even religious. This phenomenon increases the country's already very heavy economic and health burdens through the burden of communicable and nutritional diseases. They lead to dissension in the population, allow charlatans to manipulate the population, reduce the population's confidence in the national health system, oppose the population to the political authorities and increase the East-West geopolitical divide in the country.

It was necessary to start research, first to understand what was really happening and then to try to find a valid scientific response to secure the population. The flow of patients, which was initially low, has increased over time so that today, not a day goes by without new cases coming from all over the country, sometimes even from outside the country.

2.2 General objective

The general objective of this research was to study the phenomenon of poisoning in the Democratic Republic of Congo and some other countries in sub-Saharan Africa.

2.3 Specific objectives

The specific objectives were to: assess the extent of the problem, determine the target population, determine the profile of patients, identify symptoms, establish the route of patients until their arrival at the Toxicology Department, evaluate traditional and modern means of control, study the possible influence of HIV, investigate the factors involved, generate hypotheses on the real identity of the Karuho phenomenon and propose appropriate solutions.

2.4 Methodology

2.4.1 Study population

The study population included all patients who, as mentioned above, have been coming to the Toxicology Department of the University of Kinshasa since 1990, for better care.

2.4.2 Study site

The headquarters of the study was the Toxicology Department of the University of Kinshasa. The analysis of biological parameters was carried out at the Biochemistry Laboratory of the Faculty of Pharmaceutical Sciences of the University of Kinshasa. Medical examinations were carried out in specialized laboratories of hospitals, when the patients' pockets allowed it.

2.4.3 Methods

2.4.3.1 Data collection

Data collection was done by means of a questionnaire. However, listening to patients was a golden rule because it was essential to use patients as partners in this research.

2.4.3.2 Study variables

The variables of interest were: age, sex, marital status, education, province or country of origin, residence, nature and circumstances of onset of symptoms, medical itinerary before arrival at the Toxicology Department, testing, diagnosis and traditional treatments, test, diagnosis and modern treatments, medical history, chronic diseases: diabetes, hypertension, gastralgia and others, opinion on "poisonings", opinion on the poison Karuho: origin, nature, mechanism of action, psychological state of the patient and the family members, who referred them to the Toxicology Department, common food: (meat, fish, chicken, vegetables, fruits and dairy products (milk, curd, cheese, yogurt, beans, ...), common drinks: (water, sparkling water, alcohol (beer, wine and liquors), sugary soft drinks, non-alcoholic beer, traditional drinks and natural fruit juice.

2.4.3.3 Toxicological screening

The toxicological screening was conducted according to the "Basic Analytical Toxicology" of R.J. Flanagan et al., published in 2003 by the World Health Organization, in collaboration with the United Nations Environment Programme and the International Labour Organization, which offers researchers in developing countries simple analytical techniques but highly effective, able to solve complex toxicological problems with reduced material and financial resources. Thus, toxicological screening was carried out by urine tests, thin-layer chromatography on mini-plates and ultraviolet spectrophotometry [10, 11].

2.4.3.4 Biological parameters

The biological parameters examined were: haemoglobin, white-blood cell formula, fasting blood glucose, sedimentation rate, alanine aminotransferase, aspartate aminotransferase, urea, creatinine, thick gout, dimers, typhoid fever and *Helicobacter pylori.*

2.4.3.5 Medical examinations

The medical examinations were as follows: electrocardiogram, cardiac ultrasound, abdominal ultrasound, renal ecography, electroencephalogram, spirometer and CT scanner.

2.4.3.6 Data interpretation

In accordance with the literature, data interpretation used toxicoepidemiology. The world toxicological history informs that the Congolese are not the only ones or the first to face an unknown danger, exciting their imagination. Indeed, leprosy was considered a curse, the intoxication of Minamata Bay as a bad fate and for the Fire of Saint Anthony, the sick were accused of witchcraft. Toxicology also indicates that epidemiology has been the appropriate weapon for solving toxicological puzzles, including that of toxic cancer [12–19].

This is why our research used toxicoepidemiology in the face of imaginary poisonings in DR Congo. It was supplemented by induction inference, allowing to go from the particular to the general, as well as by Mill's criteria, to identify the causes of pathologies, and explain their distribution within the population and Bloom's taxonomy, a tool of pedagogy by objective which, by a logical deduction, makes it possible to create new knowledge from a first simple knowledge [20, 21].

2.5 Results

The toxicological screening was negative for most of the patients. **Table 1** shows that of the 1572 patients who were examined, 1430 (90.7%) were negative. The 142 (9.3%) patients who tested positive were for the paracetamol that these patients were taking to combat stomach pain. *Helicobacter pylori* was positive in all patients with a score of 100%. Iron deficiency anemia was identified in 95 (6%) patients. The liver parameters aspartate-amino-transferase (ASAT) as well as alanine-amino-transferase

Variables	Patients	Percentages
Population of study		
Unmarried	377	24
Married	1084	69
Formerly married	110	7
Total	1572	100
Age		
0–5	12	0.8
6–20	217	13.8
21–50	1183	75.2
More than 50	160	10.2
Total	1572	100
Gender		
Male	1038	66
Female	534	33.9
Residence		
Kinshasa	1037	66
Other provinces	487	31
Other countries	48	3
Total	1572	100
Education		
No education	172	11
Primary	188	12
High	408	26
Higher	801	51
Total	1572	100
Patients progression from 2005 to 2023		
2005–2016	402	25.5
2017	186	11.8
2018	220	13.9
2019	245	15.5
2020–2021	53	3.3
2022	124	7.8
2023	342	21.7
Total	1572	100
Toxicological screening		
Negative	1430	90.7
Positive	142	9.3
Helicobacter pylori		

Variables	Patients	Percentages
Positive	1575	100
Negative	0	0
Hemoglobin		
Normal	1477	94
Anormal	95	6
Aspartate aminotransferase (ASAT)		
Normal	1382	87.8
Anormal	193	12.2
Alanine aminotransferase (ALAT)		
Normal	1387	88.1
Anormal	188	11.9
Creatinin		
Normal	1496	95
Anormal	79	5
Urea		
Normal	1512	96
Anormal	63	4

Comments: *The study was carried out from July 2005 to May 2023 on a total number of 1572 patients distributed as follows: 347 (24%) single, 1084 (92%) married and 110 (7%) widowed. The age of the majority of respondents ranges from 21 to 50 years, with 1183 (75.2%) sick. There were 12 (0.8%) children aged under 5 years. There were more men: 1038 (66%) compared to 534 (34%) women. While at the beginning, the patients only came from the North-East of the country, mainly from the city of Goma, the city of Kinshasa, the most populous province of DR Congo, took the lead with 1037 (66%) sick. A total of 48 (3%) patients came from abroad, from Cameroon and the Republic of Congo. In terms of education, academics come first with 801 (51%) sick people. The number of patients was low at the beginning with an average rate of 33 (2.05%) patients per year during the first 12 years. Then it started to increase: 186 (11.8%) in 2017, 220 (13.9%) in 2018 and 245 (15.5%) in 2019. In 2020 and 2021 the number fell to 53 (3.3%) for both years due to COVID-19 infection. It then increased to 124 (7.8%) patients in 2022 and 342 (21.7%) patients in 2023, until May.*

Table 1.
Results of variables of interest.

(ALAT) were normal in most cases, 1382 (87.8%) and 1387 (88.1%) respectively. Most cases of abnormal ASAT and ALAT were due to the presence of excess paracetamol. Urinary parameters, creatinine and urea were also normal in most cases, i.e. 1496 (95%) for creatinine and 1512 (96%) for urea. The disruption of renal parameters most often came from the uncontrolled treatments that patients received during their visit to traditional practitioners before their arrival at the Toxicology Department.

2.6 *Helicobacter pylori* role

It was in 2010 that the unexpected discovery of *Helicobacter pylori* as the cause of suspected poisoning in DR Congo was established. It all started with a young doctor from a public company in the city of Kinshasa who recommended a patient suspected of poisoning, presenting the same many and singular symptoms as the others who came to the Toxicology Department. However, this patient also had recurrent iron deficiency anemia requiring repeated blood transfusions. The young doctor who had been our toxicology student at the Faculty of Medicine of the University of Kinshasa thought that the patient could be poisoned with lead.

Lead, is indeed a very dangerous toxic of the group of heavy metals or metal trace elements, which can cause recurrent iron deficiency anemia in humans. Indeed, it inhibits the enzyme "ALAD" (deltaminolevulinic acid), which allows the conversion of porphyrin into hemoglobin, which leads to the accumulation of porphyrins in the blood. It also opposes the incorporation of iron at the level of protoporphyrin and weakens red blood cells, thus shortening their average lifespan [22–24].

Fortunately, like some other cumulative toxicants, lead poisoning already manifests itself during the preclinical phase, by three very early warning signs of poisoning. These are Burton's line, black stool staining and accumulation of coproporphyrin in urine. The patient did not have Burton's line, which is a simple but significant gray line visible at the base of the gums, attesting to the deposit of dental lead. His stools were not black either. In addition, analyses of urinary coproporphyrin and lead were carried out with a visible spectrophotometer using the Schwartz method, Zieve and Watson for coproporphyrin and analysis at the wavelength of 515 nm, after complexation with dithizone in chloroform for lead, also gave negative results [25–27].

Fortunately, the literature on *Helicobacter pylori* reminded us that, since 1993, *Helicobacter pylori* had been implicated in several cases of unexplained iron deficiency anemia. It seemed useful to us at any chance to explore this new path after that of lead [28–31].

2.7 Acceptance into international conferences

Very quickly, this new track, which seemed very uncredible at first, turned out to be the right one, as evidenced by our results, which were accepted in international journals and validated in several of the following international forums:

- "9th International Symposium on Recent Advances in Environmental Health Research, Jackson State University, USA". Poster presentation: "Helicobacter pylori responsible of poisoning suspicion in the democratic republic of Congo: about 56 cases".

- 2016, "3rd Euro-Global Experts Meeting on Medical Case Reports (Euro Case Reports 2016), June 30-July 2, Valencia, Spain". Oral presentation:

  "Surprising unknown H. pylori epidemic in the Democratic Republic of the Congo".

- 2017, "5th European Conference on Clinical and Medical Case reports, September 7-8, 2017, Paris, France". One oral and three following poster presentations:

Oral presentation: "Meanders of an atypical research work on Helicobacter pylori in the Democratic Republic of the Congo: influence of HIV and other factors and study of some interesting cases".

Tree poster presentations:

"Profile of Helicobacter pylori patients received at the laboratory of Toxicology of the University of Kinshasa from July 2016 to July 2017".

"Opinion of population of Kinshasa City on Helicobacter pylori phenomenon responsible of numerous extra-digestive pathologies in DR Congo".

"About the management of Helicobacter pylori infection expressing numerous extra-digestive pathologies in DR Congo".

- 2017, "7th International Conference on Predictive, Preventive and Personalized Medicine & Molecular Diagnostics, September 14-15, 2017, Edinburgh, Scotland".

  E-Poster presentation: "Helicobacter pylori digestive and extra-digestive pathologies collected in the Democratic Republic of the Congo".

- 2018, "Joint Pharmaceutical conference Democratic Republic of Congo Kinshasa and Republic of Congo Brazzaville, at Pointe Noire city": Oral Presentation: "Karuho poison and Helicobacter pylori: Two features, One issue, One solution".

- 2018, "Joint Event on International Conference on Pharmaceutics and Novel Drug Delivery Systems & 19th International Conference on Cellular and Molecular Medicine & 19th Annual Congress on Psychiatry and Psychiatric Disorders, held in Narita, Japan".

  "Toxicological aspects of Helicobacter pylori infection established in Democratic Republic of the Congo consecutively to massive poisoning suspicions all over the country".

- 2018, "7th International Conference on Predictive, Preventive and Personalized Medicine & Molecular Diagnostics October 26-27, 2018, Boston, USA". Oral presentation: "Successful toxicological Helicobacter pylori infection treatment conducted in a male Congolese patient with severe hemoglobin deficiency in the Democratic Republic of the Congo".

- 2019, " 2nd world congress and expo on Toxicology and Pharmacology" , October 28-29, Rome, Italy.

  Oral presentation: "Unexpcted interesting Toxicological trends in Helicobacter pylori infection in Democratic Republic of Congo, A case report" .

- 2019, "2nd world Congress an Expo on Dentistry and Oral Health", October 30-31, 2019, Rome, Italy".

  Oral presentation: "Impact of Helicobacter pylori intoxication in Throat, Mouth, Eyes and Face Skin Health in the Democratic Republic of Congo".

2.8 Digestive and extra-digestive symptoms collected from patients

Several symptoms have been observed during the study. These symptoms collected from patients are presented in **Table 2**.

Digestive symptoms	General symptoms	Nervous symptoms
• Heat in the stomach that can radiate to the chest • Strong abdominal pain • Belly buzzing • Dry throat • Burning of the tongue • Dry lips • Taste of chili on the lips • Bitter or bland taste of food and drink • Hyper-salivation • Nausea • Vomiting • Regurgitation • Hiccups • Bloody sputum • Constipation • Belly bloating • Increased pH and viscosity of saliva: saliva becomes alkaline and sticky • Sensation of something in the throat	• Pronounced weight loss • Strong heat in other parts of the body, even on the feet • Hyperthermia • Heavy sweating • Tingling and tingling • Skin blackening and signs of early aging • General fatigue • Sexual weakness • Heart palpitations • Choking and shortness of breath • Difficult breathing • Hormonal disorders • Anemia • Skin allergies • Swelling of the feet • Dry cough • Lack of appetite • Oxygen desaturation • Deposition of ammonium carbonate in the lungs	• Dizziness and feeling high • Imbalance • Frequent and throbbing headaches • Sensation of something moving in the head • Blurred vision • Ringing in the ears • Intermittent tremors of legs and hands • Memory disturbance with frequent forgetfulness • Mental confusion • Strong desire to sleep with sometimes loss of consciousness, mental confusion and temporary amnesia • Visual hallucinations • Electroencephalogram disruption • Tingling and tickling • Frequent insomnia

Comments: *The most common symptoms are constipation, weight loss, loss of appetite, stomach pain and bloating. Then comes gas in the stomach, heat that can spread throughout the body, heavy sweating, heart palpitations, dry mouth and throat, dry cough, sputum, burning of the tongue, small sores in the mouth, bland, spicy or bitter taste, stuffy or runny nose, ear pain, blurred vision and darkening of the skin. Dizziness, headache, insomnia, memory disturbance, asthenia, sexual weakness, back pain, pain, heat or swelling of the legs, itching, cramps in the feet and hands, disturbance of menstruation and itching of the private parts in women. Difficulty breathing, shortness of breath, premature aging, dehydration, hypovolemia, allergy, seizures, headaches, fever, coma and death. Abundant nausea and vomiting which can also lead to death.*

Table 2.
Symptoms collected from patients.

3. Pathophysiology

3.1 Description

Helicobacter pylori appears to be under the control of blood pH which modulates the acid-base balance of the body. When the pH of the blood is normal, the amount of acid in the stomach is normal too. *Helicobacter pylori* stays then in the gastric mucosa, protected by gastric mucus, for as long as necessary, without ever harming its host.

When the pH of the blood increases, gastric acidity decreases as a result of the action of bicarbonate. This occurs when the body is in a state of chronic respiratory acidosis or compensated respiratory acidosis. Respiratory acidosis is a primitive increase in the amount of carbon dioxide in the blood. When bicarbonate increases to compensate for this excess carbon dioxide, it is called chronic respiratory acidosis or compensated respiratory acidosis.

Blood pH is normally low but can also be close to normal. Helicobacter takes advantage of this situation of chronic acidosis to consolidate its position in the gastric mucosa by attaching more firmly to the epithelial cells of the gastric mucosa and activating certain virulence genes such as cagA and vacA that govern stomach inflammation and cancer genesis. It also secretes cytotoxins and mucolytic enzymes that can damage gastric epithelial cells and promote pathogenesis. Aggression of the mucus barrier can lead to gastritis, peptic ulcer, gastric cancer or gastric lymphoma.

When, on the other hand, the pH of the blood decreases, which happens especially in this case, where there is sudden inhalation of atmospheric air rich in carbon dioxide, gastric acidity increases. There is acute respiratory acidosis. Respiratory acidosis is acute when the increase in carbon dioxide is not accompanied by a concomitant increase in bicarbonate, compensating for the excess carbon dioxide. *Helicobacter pylori* faces excess gastric acidity. In this case, it naturally uses its urease enzyme to produce carbon dioxide and ammonia that can protect it from this excess acidity [32–34].

Normally, after their production, both gases are eliminated in the stool in liquid form. But, in case of respiratory acidosis that leads to acidification of the intestinal environment, modifying the bacterial flora and disrupting digestion, strong constipation occurs in patients. Constipation can also be a side effect of respiratory acidosis, as excess carbon dioxide can reduce intestinal peristalsis and promote stool retention. Following this constipation, gas accumulates in the stomach and intestines. There is bloating and appetite is disturbed, leading to weight loss. The pressure of bloating causes gases to rise along the oesophagus with strong heat that burns the throat, mouth, nose, ears, brain and lungs. Once in the lungs, carbon dioxide and ammonia gas generate another highly caustic toxicant, ammonium carbonate, before passing into the blood through the pulmonary alveoli. Ammonium carbonate causes dry cough, sputum, chest heaviness and heart palpitations. All these symptoms are felt by our patients. Ammonium carbonate could also cause pulmonary fibrosis and, even, lung cancer. Ammonia is a very violent gas that can cause obstruction of the upper pulmonary tract and even pulmonary oedema. It can also solubilize in mucosal water to form ammonium hydroxide, a very strong and very caustic base and hydroxyl ions in an exothermic reaction, releasing a strong heat that patients can hardly tolerate [35–39].

There is thus first environmental poisoning, by nasal inhalation of atmospheric carbon dioxide, leading to acute respiratory acidosis. To this first poisoning is added a second one, caused by ammonia and carbon gases produced by *Helicobacter pylori* in the stomach. Both gases also reach the lungs but, through the larynx and not through the nose. This is a special internal inhalation poisoning. Similar intoxication, by internal inhalation, is described in the literature. It concerns in particular ruminant bovains fed, at the end of the 70s, with large quantities of urea. This bovine poisoning lends credence to our discovery of *Helicobacter pylori* poisoning, as both involve the urease enzyme, producing carbon dioxide and ammonia from urea, reaching the lungs by internal inhalation [40–45].

If carbon dioxide and ammonia are inhaled at the same time, the pH of the blood may vary depending on the concentration and duration of exposure to the gases. Carbon dioxide dissolves in the blood and forms carbonic acid, which lowers the pH of the blood (respiratory acidosis). Ammonia dissolves in water in the lining of the respiratory tract and increases the pH of the blood (respiratory alkalosis).

Both gases are very hot and, as said above, they burn the mucous membranes very strongly starting with the upper nasal and pulmonary mucous membranes, before extending to the mucous membranes of the other parts of the body. With regard to carbon dioxide, in 1986, the limnic eruption at Lake Nyos, Cameroon, in the English-speaking North-West region, allowed the world to discover the highly calorific properties of carbon dioxide. More than 1700 people died in this natural disaster but above all, most of the victims had deep burns that were observed for the first time and that were recognized as caused by carbon dioxide [46–48].

The consequence of this kind of internal boiler is heavy perspiration, especially during the night, when the patient is sleeping. This heavy perspiration has as a corollary, a strong dehydration that affects all parts of the body, among others: the skin, especially that of the face, all mucous membranes, especially oral and ones, blood volume (hypovolemia), saliva and darkening of the skin. If dehydration reaches the intracellular level, convulsions, headache, high fever, coma and death are noted [49, 50].

In this regard, here is the situation experienced by a patient for a year, from April 2019 to May 2020, commented by his daughter:

- Dad began his ordeal on April 7, 2019, with small convulsions, as if he were epileptic. The next day, a high fever appeared. The thermometer reached up to 39.40°C. Dad was committed to the hospital for a month and every day a high fever was present. He was sweating and shivering profusely. The traditional saliva test performed by a tradipratician smuggled into the hospital by the family came back positive. The family then took Dad out, claiming lack of means. The tradipratician followed us home. Two days after the traditional treatment began, Dad suddenly went into a coma. It took 4 days of intensive care in the hospital for Dad to come back to life. Sometime later, he flew to Europe for treatment. Here too, a surprise awaited him but still happier although really unexpected. Indeed, 3 weeks later, while the doctors were still doing their investigations, suddenly, the fever stopped on its own without any treatment. Dad was asked to remain at the doctors' disposal until the fever resumed. He would have liked to do it but, another surprise, came to upset everything, the COVID-19 epidemic. In December 2019, Papa had to leave Europe in a hurry to return to Kinshasa. In January 2020, another surprise, this one unfortunate, emerged; the resumption of a fever, as strong as before his departure to Europe. Dad was committed to another hospital where he spent 4 months without the slightest relief! Eventually, he had to leave the hospital and was taken home with his fever. He could no longer stand up and eat. His weight loss had reached frightening proportions. A traditional healer was brought in once again. The traditional test turned out once again positive, while in the hospital it had been thought to attribute this fever to COVID-19. The treatment of the new tradipratician brought no relief either.

This case was very helpful. First, the fever was stopped by eliminating gas with strong adsorbents and laxatives and intensive oral rehydration. Secondly, it was then possible, thanks to Mill's criteria, to establish the role of carbon dioxide and ammonia released by *Helicobacter pylori* in the stomach, in the phenomenon of suspected poisoning in DR Congo. On the other hand, it has been possible, still thanks to Mill's criteria, to determine environmental pollution as the factor present in Kinshasa and managed in Europe, responsible for fever, and activating factor of *Helicobacter pylori*, as already described in our presentations at international conferences as well as in our publications. One of our publications even reported the results of an autopsy performed on one of our deceased patients which showed the swelling of the intestines and stomach, as well as the burning of the brain, lungs and feet by gas. The nature of these gases is beyond doubt since the signs of asphyxiation by carbon dioxide were clearly reported: blackened nails and toes, red eyes and self-bite of the tongue (**Figures 1–6**) [51].

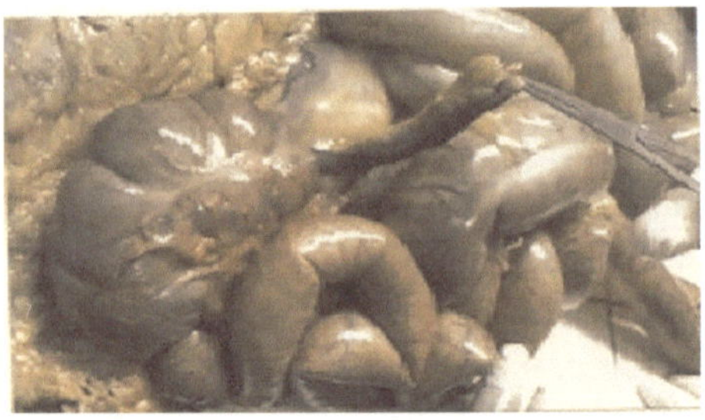

Figure 1.
Gut distending photo Forensic Medicine Kinshasa.

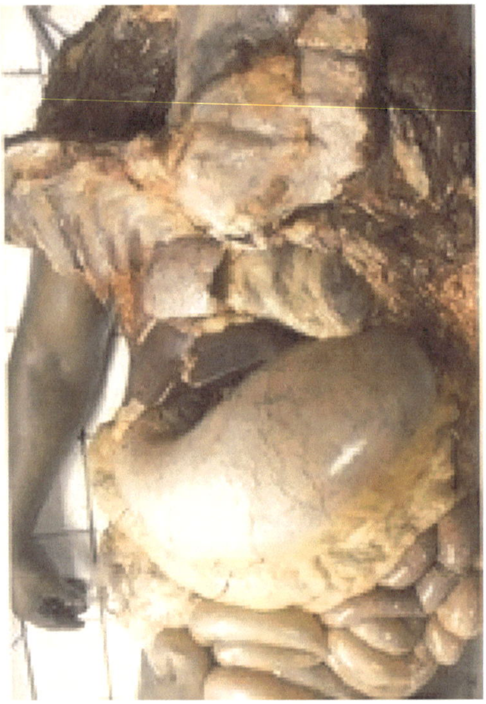

Figure 2.
Stomach distending photo Forensic Medicine Institute/Kinshasa.

The severe dehydration and alkalinization of saliva by ammonia gas scientifically justify the traditional test of "poisoning" practiced by traditional healers on the saliva of patients.

In the throat, there is dryness and sputum that can be bloody [45]. Patients sometimes have a sensation of something in the throat, which makes breathing difficult, with shortness of breath and suffocation at night. The voice can become hoarse, so singing and, even speaking, becomes difficult. Sometimes the voice even goes out. In case of tooth decay, the tooth can sometimes break or crumble on its own, because of the heat excreted by the gases in the mouth.

The bitter taste of food and drink is common among sick people. This symptom is also related to the high heat of the gases in the mouth, which here burn the taste buds

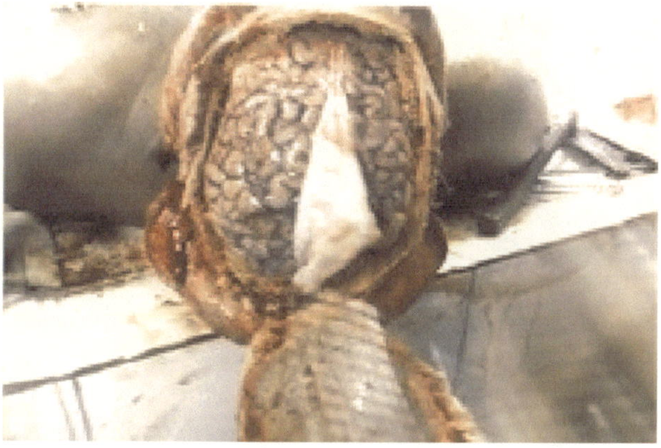

Figure 3.
Brain congestion photo Forensic Medicine Institute/Kinshasa.

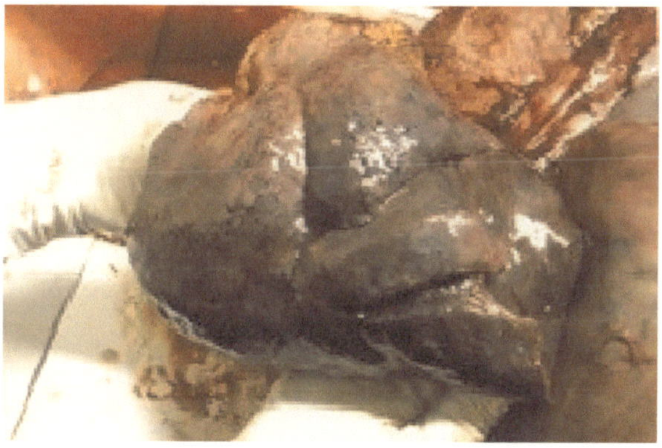

Figure 4.
Right lung congestion photo Forensic Medicine Institute/Kinshasa.

of the tongue. It is a reason for dissension among the population. Indeed, it would seem to be the proof of poisoning and also the indication of the poisoner. Here are a few examples.

- My cross began during a ceremony organized within our Church between our Pastor and the new Pastor who came to replace him, said Mr. Josué, a fervent member of one of the many revival churches in the city of Kinshasa. I let myself be trapped like a child. Indeed, I knew well that our Pastor did not love me; and that he considered me responsible for the strong reactions of the members of our community against him which resulted in his departure! He even attacked me in some of his sermons. Despite all this, I agreed to be served first and from the first bites I immediately felt a strong bitterness in my mouth, as if I had a quinine tablet in my mouth! I ran to spit everything in the toilet but it was too late.

- Last Saturday, says Mrs. Esperance, I went to visit a friend and she offered me food. Until then, everything was normal. But when it was time to drink water, I

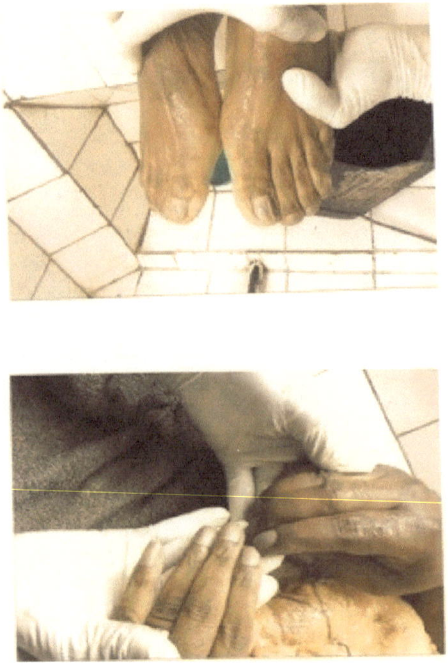

Figure 5.
Fingers and toes cyanosis photo Forensic Medicine Institute/Kinshasa.

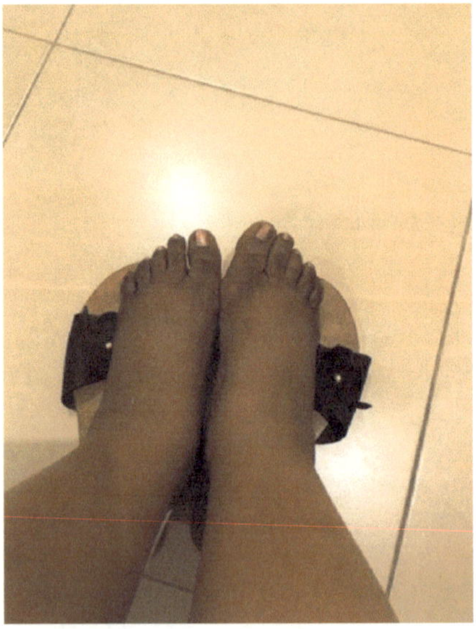

Figure 6.
Feet swelling photo Shafali/Kinshasa. Comments: ***Figures 1–6*** *are taken from one of our publications published in 2018. It reports the results of an autopsy carried out at the Institute of Forensic Medicine of the Kinshasa General Hospital, after a suspicious death of a patient known to have chronic gastritis to* Helicobacter pylori. *This autopsy showed various abnormalities as follows: swelling of the intestines, swelling of the stomach, cerebral congestion, congestion of the lungs, cyanosis of the lips, fingers and toes, biting of the tongue, pallor of the palms of the hands and pallor of the soles of the feet, cardiomegaly, red colouring of the eyes, nosebleeds, gastric bleeding and asphyxia by carbon dioxide. All these anomalies lend credibility to the double intoxication by carbon dioxide and ammonia presented in this chapter.*

felt that it was very bitter. Afterwards, I felt that my tongue was burned as if I had drunk water that was too hot and yet it was not. My lips were also burning, as if chili pepper had been applied to them. That's how mean people can be!

Flu, angina and colds are regular. The nose is often stuffy. Sinusitis is often diagnosed in many of these patients. Hot gases, as said above, spare no part of the body. Vision is often blurred even if the person wears medical glasses. And cases of double cataracts are common. The ears ring, hiss, become painful or even sometimes, sometimes hearing decreases.

Hot gases reach the brain and cause dizziness, headaches, insomnia, imbalance and even memory disturbance. This is observed by frequent forgetfulness even for young patients. Even worse, the person sometimes becomes unable to continue his sentence because he forgets the beginning and loses the thread of ideas. It takes a while for him sometimes to find himself or someone has to help him. Insomnia is often strong, as well as sometimes, visual hallucinations, loss of consciousness, mental confusion, vision and hearing disorders and intermittent tremors of the legs and hands! Some patients sometimes feel discomfort in the head, difficult to define. Some others sometimes even feel a kind of temporary madness. The electroencephalogram is often disturbed.

Fatigue is almost permanent. There is drowsiness during the day. There is also strong sexual weakness in both men and women. Sexual strength and desire decrease. Some women become frigid. Sexual weakness leads to discord in homes and sometimes even leads to divorce.

Fatigue is caused by the attack of gases on the brain combined with oxygen desaturation which is common in almost all patients, and which also explains the sexual weakness that occurs even in young people still in their twenties. Lack of oxygen also leads to metabolic acidosis. The organic acids generated participate in the melting of muscles and the development of cramps in the hands and feet.

There is also itching, swelling of the legs, tingling in the legs and arms, heat or pain under the soles of the feet, allergies, hypertension and diabetic crises. Finally, there are signs of early aging: the skin darkens, the face becomes dry and wrinkled, the gait is hesitant, the hands or fingers sometimes tremble and there is an imbalance when walking or even when you suddenly stand.

3.2 Pathophysiological scheme of *Helicobacter pylori* poisoning

See **Figure** 7.

4. New innovative hypotheses

Helicobacter pylori is widespread throughout the world, colonizing more than half of the world's population. In 80% of cases, the infection is asymptomatic. Symptoms of infection are observed in only 20% of patients and they mainly include acute gastritis, chronic gastritis, gastric ulcer and gastric cancer. Gastric cancer follows gastric ulcer disease and occurs in a small proportion of 1–3% of cases of gastric ulcer disease.

Despite the low frequency of stomach cancer linked to *Helicobacter pylori*, it is one of the deadliest cancers in the world and *Helicobacter pylori* infection is categorized as a class one carcinogen. The eradication of *Helicobacter pylori* in patients with gastric ulcers should be the solution to prevent this cancer. Unfortunately, *Helicobacter pylori*

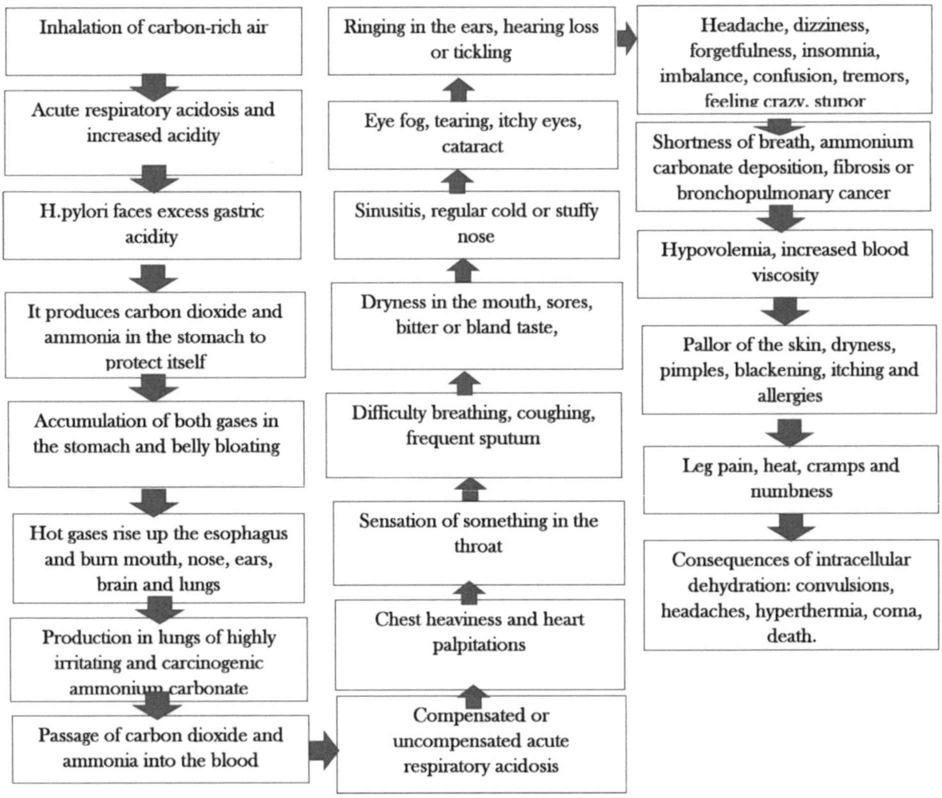

Figure 7.
Physiological scheme of Helicobacter pylori *poisoning.*

is one of the most resistant bacteria in the world. It is resistant to various treatments, including quadruple therapy, currently used, after tritherapy.

New treatment principles are therefore necessary.

Our research comes at the right time in this regard. Indeed, it reveals a new face of *Helicobacter pylori* infection, previously unknown, which states that *Helicobacter pylori* is sensitive to environmental pollution in the same way as humans. By protecting itself against this pollution, especially represented by atmospheric carbon dioxide, the bacteria cause intoxication by carbon dioxide and ammonia which is described in the present chapter and which has been considered impossible until now, in the literature.

This new face of *Helicobacter pylori* was discovered in the Democratic Republic of Congo, following the fact that any foreign person, colonized by *Helicobacter pylori*, symptomatic or asymptomatic, going to Goma and Bukavu, rich in environmental carbon dioxide released from the Nyiragongo Volcano and the Lake Kivu, develops, after a few days, the symptoms of carbon dioxide and ammonia poisoning described in this chapter, which the population until now considers to be massive poisonings perpetrated by evil people. These patients are valuable in our research because they attest both to the link between atmospheric pollution, urease and *Helicobacter pylori* infection, as well as that between gastritis and constipation, practically present in all of our patients.

Our research reveals that the intensity of poisoning is a function of the intensity of environmental carbon pollution. It is the latter which determines the degree of production of carbon dioxide and ammonia by *Helicobacter pylori*. The threshold at which air pollution activates the bacteria is currently in progress within our research team, by mathematical modelling. The second factor that plays a determining role in this poisoning is constipation, responsible for the accumulation of the two gases in the stomach, which allows them to rise along the oesophagus and pass into the blood through the pulmonary alveoli, as well as their distribution throughout the body.

Our research reveals that the inflammation that causes symptoms of *Helicobacter pylori* infection, from gastritis to gastric cancer, comes from the high heat accompanying the two gases released by *Helicobacter pylori* [52]. It is important to remember, in this regard, the strong inflammation produced by carbon dioxide during the limnic irruption that occurred in 1987 at Lake Nyos in Cameroon, which caused terrible burns on the victims.

Our research recommends changing the approach to combat the symptoms of *Helicobacter pylori* infection, from gastritis to gastric cancer as well as those described in this chapter. She advises not to concentrate on the bacteria but on the factors which make it dangerous: atmospheric pollution which is at the origin of the reaction of *Helicobacter pylori*, urease which allows the bacteria to react by producing gases ammonia and carbon dioxide, the ammonia and carbon dioxide gases responsible for inflammation, the cause of all the ills caused by the bacteria and, finally, strong and permanent constipation, which prevents the two gases from being eliminated in the stools in liquid form.

4.1 Air pollution

Fighting air pollution at a time when greenhouse gases, mainly carbon dioxide, are in full expansion, is not easy. For example, the Democratic Republic of Congo hosts three important natural carbon dioxide production sites: the Nyiragongo Volcano, Lake Kivu and the peatlands of the equatorial forest [53, 54]. In addition to this natural production of greenhouse gases, there is another production of gas caused by man. The situation is not different in other Saharan African countries. Intensive reforestation is therefore essential. At the same time, we encourage studies of chemical conversion of environmental carbon dioxide into a less dangerous product, undertaken throughout the world. Finally, a study of the historical behaviour of *Helicobacter pylori* infection throughout human history, in light of the discovery of the influence of greenhouse gases on this infection, would be highly useful.

4.2 Urease and antiurease

Antiurease is the best solution to deal with infection or better, *Helicobacter pylori* poisoning. In fact, it prevents the production of the two gases that generate inflammation. Many studies relating to the search for antiurease are underway throughout the world but the solution is still lacking [55–57]. Our research team has been interested in this challenge for a long time and to our great surprise, an enzyme drug, found on the market, has given incredibly satisfactory results. Unfortunately, this drug was shortly after modified by the company which had designed it and its antiurease properties had been disrupted. Contact with this firm is strongly considered to be able to carry out tests with the old formula of this product.

4.3 Constipation

Constipation is the real cause of all the problems that *Helicobacter pylori* causes in the human body. Indeed, if there is no constipation, the ammonia and carbon dioxide gases produced by *Helicobacter pylori* become liquid, and are eliminated without difficulty in the stools. The patient is then completely asymptomatic. Thus, in the absence of an antiurease, treatment of constipation is the best response against this infection. Unfortunately, this constipation is very strong. This severe constipation is due respectively to the accumulation of gases in the digestive tract which slow down intestinal transit, the concentration and fermentation of more or less dry stools in the large intestine, the disruption of macrobiota with the development of bad bacteria and sometimes the occurrence of haemorrhoids. Our research in this regard is directed towards Congolese and African medicinal plants, but also to specialists in the study of constipation throughout the world.

5. Conclusion

The link established between suspected poisoning, the environment and *Helicobacter pylori* in the Democratic Republic of Congo sheds exceptional light on *Helicobacter pylori* infection. We learn that *Helicobacter pylori* is sensitive to environmental pollution, mainly atmospheric. If this pollution exceeds a certain threshold, a disruption of intestinal transit may result, the carbon dioxide and ammonia released by *Helicobacter pylori* in the stomach can accumulate and pass into the blood through the pulmonary alveoli. If atmospheric pollution constitutes the external factor responsible for this poisoning, urease and constipation constitute the internal factors which must be combated in the same way. The application of the principles set out in this chapter could also make it possible to effectively combat or better prevent gastric cancer linked to *Helicobacter pylori*.

Our team is open to international collaborations that could allow us to obtain the financial and material resources necessary to continue our research.

Author details

Josaphat Ndelo di Phanzu*, Lievins-Corneille Mputu Malolo, Patrick Ndelo Matondo and Yannick Belo Nuapia
Toxicology Service of the University of Kinshasa, Faculty of Pharmaceutical Sciences, University of Kinshasa, Democratic Republic of the Congo

*Address all correspondence to: jos_ndelo@yahoo.fr

References

[1] Marshall B. A Brief History of the Discovery of *Helicobacter pylori*. In: *Helicobacter pylori*. Springer; 2016

[2] Charitos IA, D'Agostino D, Topi S, Bottalico L. 40 years of *Helicobacter pylori*: A revolution in biomedical thought. Gastroenterology Insights. 2021. Available from: mdpi.com

[3] Buzás GM. History of the discovery of *Helicobacter pylori*. Orvostorteneti Kozlemenyek. 2004. Available from: europepmc.org

[4] Ivanova. The history of the discovery of the *Helicobacter pylori*. Terapevticheskii. 2022. Available from: ter-arkhiv.ru

[5] Goodwin CS, Mendall MM, Northfield TC. *Helicobacter pylori* infection. The Lancet. 1997. Available from: thelancet.com

[6] Crowe SE. *Helicobacter pylori* infection. New England Journal of Medicine. 2019

[7] Mwabi AN, Ntakarutimana V, Bisimwa GB. Poisoning investigations in the City of Bukavu and the effects of antidotes administered by traditional healers. International Journal of Innovative Science and Research Technology. 2020;5(2):2002-2011. Available from: ijisrt.com

[8] Kaboru BB, Namegabe EN. Geographical, health systems' and sociocultural patterns of TB/HIV co-infected patients' health seeking behavior in a conflict affected setting: The case of eastern Democratic Republic of Congo. Journal of Community Medicine and Health Education. 2013. Available from: diva-portal.org

[9] Kyolo SK, Bbosa GS, Odda J, Lubeg AM. Toxicity profile of Karuho Poison on the brain of Wistar Albino rats. Neuroscience and Medicine. 2018. Available from: articlearchives.org

[10] Flanagan RJ, Braithwaite RA, Brown SS, Widdop B. Basic Analytical Toxicology. 1995. Available from: apps.who.int

[11] Flanagan RJ, Taylor AA, Watson ID, Whelpton. Fundamentals of Analytical Toxicology. 2008. Available from: books.google.com

[12] Joubert B, Sebata P. The role of prospective epidemiology in the establishment of a toxicology service for a developing community. South African Medical Journal. 1982. Available from: journals.co.za

[13] Andrew E, Irestedt B, Hurri T, Jacobsen P. Mortality and morbidity of poisonings in the Nordic countries in 2002. Clinical Toxicology. 2008

[14] Piekarska-Wijatkowska A, Czyzewska S, Kotwica M, Krakowiak A. Epidemiology of acute poisonings during 2002-2011 in toxicology unit; Department of Occupational Medicine and Toxicology, Nofer Institute of Occupational Medicine. Przegląd Lekarski. 2013. Available from: europepmc.org

[15] Une maladie de la pollution : Minamata. Ui J, Janon M. Esprit, 1940, 477-489. 1973.

[16] Ui J, Janin M. Esprit (1940-). JSTOR. 1973

[17] Vassallo L. L'adoption de la Convention de Minamata, ou la longue marche vers un instrument international

juridiquement contraignant sur le mercure. Revue Juridique de l'Environnement. 2013. Available from: cairn.info

[18] Battin J. Le feu Saint-Antoine ou ergotisme gangreneux et son iconographie médiévale. Histoire des Sciences Médicales. 2010. Available from: biusante.parisdescartes.fr

[19] McElveen JC Jr, Eddy PS. Cancer and toxic substances: The problem of causation and the use of epidemiology. Cleveland State Law Review. 1984

[20] MacHardy WE, Gadoury DM. A revision of Mills' s criteria for predicting apple scab infection periods. Phytopathology. 1989. Available from: apsnet.org

[21] Forehand M. Bloom's taxonomy: Original and revised. In: Emerging Perspectives on Learning, Teaching and Technology. 2005;(8):41-44. Available from: cmapspublic3.ihmc.us

[22] Karita K, Yano E, Dakeishi M, Iwata T, Katsuyuki M. Benchmark dose of lead inducing anemia at the workplace. Risk Analysis: An International Journal. Wiley Online Library. 2005

[23] Schwartz J, Landrigan PJ, Baker EL, Orenstein WA, Lindern IHV. Lead-induced anemia: Dose-response relationships and evidence for a threshold. American Journal of Public Health. 1990. Available from: ajph.aphapublications.org

[24] Hsieh NH, Chung SH, Chen SC, Chen WY, Cheng YH, Lin YJ, et al. Anemia risk in relation to lead exposure in lead-related manufacturing. BMC Public Health. Springer. 2017

[25] Pearce JMS. Burton's line in lead poisoning. European Neurology. 2007. Available from: karger.com

[26] Camuglia JE, Grigoriadis G, Gilfillan CP. Lead poisoning and Burton's line. The Medical Journal of Austaulia. 2008. Available from: mja.com.au

[27] Aziz MA, Schwartz S, Watson CJ. Studies of coproporphyrin. VII. Adaptation of the Eriksen paper chromatographic method to the quantitative analysis of the isomers in normal human urine. The Journal of Laboratory and Clinical Medicine. 1964. Available from: translationalres.com

[28] *Helicobacter pylori* Infection in Pernicious Anemia: A Prospective Controlled Study, TL Fong, CP Dooley, M Dehesa, H Cohen, R Carmel Gastroenterology, 1991

[29] Dufour C, Brisigotti M, Fabretti G, Luxardo P, Mori PG, Barabino A. *Helicobacter pylori* gastric infection and sideropenic refractory anemia. Journal of Pediatric Gastroenterology and Nutrition. 1993. Available from: journals.lww.com

[30] Wenzhen Y, Yumin L, Kehu Y, Bin M, Quanlin G, Donghai W, et al. Iron deficiency anemia in *Helicobacter pylori* infection: Meta-analysis of randomized controlled trials. Scandinavian Journal of Gastroenterology. 2010

[31] Lupu A, Miron IC, Cianga AL, Cernomaz AT, Lupu VV, Munteanu D, et al. The relationship between anemia and *Helicobacter pylori* infection in children. Children. 2022. Available from: mdpi.com

[32] Martoft L, Stødkilde-Jørgensen H, Forslid A. CO_2 induced acute respiratory acidosis and brain tissue intracellular pH: A 31P NMR study in swine. Laboratory Animals. 2003. Available from: journals.sagepub.com

[33] Testud F. Dioxyde de carbone. EMC–Pathologie Professionnelle et de l'Environnement. 2010. Available from: researchgate.net

[34] Sakhraoui PR. Troubles de l'équilibre acido-basique. Available from: univ.ency-education.com

[35] Yeh JT, Resnik KP, Rygle K, Pennline HW. Semi-batch absorption and regeneration studies for CO_2 capture by aqueous ammonia. Fuel Processing Technology. 2005

[36] Dasarathy S, Mookerjee RP, Rackayova V. Ammonia toxicity: From head to toe? Metabolic Brain Disease. 2017

[37] Close LG, Catlin FI, Cohn AM. Acute and chronic effects of ammonia burns of the respiratory tract. Archives of Otolaryngology. 1980. Available from: jamanetwork.com

[38] Rabinowitz PM, Siegel MD. Acute inhalation injury. Clinics in Chest Medicine. 2002. Available from: chestmed.theclinics.com

[39] Gorguner M, Akgun M. Acute inhalation injury. The Eurasian Journal of Medicine. 2010. Available from: ncbi.nlm.nih.gov

[40] Word JD, Martin LC, Williams DL. Urea toxicity studies in the bovine. Journal of Animal Science. 1969. Available from: academic.oup.com

[41] Boucard A. Intoxication par l'urée chez les bovins: Analyse de la base de données du CAPAE-OUEST. 2023. Available from: oniris.hal.science

[42] Austin J. Urea toxicity and its prevention. In: Urea as a Protein Supplement. Elsevier; 1967

[43] Rob O. Intoxication of cows after feeding urea. Veterinarstvi. 1960. Available from: cabdirect.org

[44] Hintz HF, Lowe JE, Clifford AJ, Visek WJ. Ammonia intoxication resulting from urea ingestion by ponies. Journal of the American Veterinary Medical Association. 1970. Available from: cabdirect.org

[45] Ndelo-di-Phanzu J et al. Impact of *Helicobacter pylori* intoxication in throat, mouth, eyes and face skin health in the Democratic Republic of Congo. EC Pharmacology and Toxicology. 2019;7(7)

[46] Kling GW, Clark MA, Wagner GN, Compton HR, Humphrey AL, Devine JD, et al. The 1986 lake nyos gas disaster in Cameroon, west Africa. Science. 1987. Available from: science.org

[47] Freeth SJ. The lake Nyos gas disaster. In: Natural Hazards in West and Central Africa. Springer; 1992

[48] Baxter PJ, Kapila M, Mfonfu D. Lake Nyos disaster, Cameroon, 1986: The medical effects of large scale emission of carbon dioxide? British Medical Journal. 1989. Available from: bmj.com

[49] Araki Y, Ando S. Urea, amino acid and ammonia in human sweat. The Japanese Journal of Physiology. 1952. Available from: jstage.jst.go.jp

[50] Cheuvront SN, Kenefick RW. Dehydration: Physiology, assessment, and performance effects. Comprehensive Physiology. 2011

[51] Ndelo-di-Phanzu MML, Ndelo Matondo P, Nuapia Y, Mbendi Nsukini J. Meanders of an atypical research work on *Helicobacter pylori* in the Democratic Republic of Congo: Influence of HIV and some other factors and study of some

interesting cases. Pharmacogenomics and Pharmacoproteomics. 2018;**9**:1. DOI: 10.4172/2153-0645.1000176

[52] Bullard RW. Effects of carbon dioxide inhalation on sweating. Journal of Applied Physiology. 1964. Available from: journals.physiology.org

[53] Fatoyinbo L. Vast peatlands found in the Congo Basin. Nature. 2017. Available from: nature.com

[54] Sonwa DJ, Bambuta JJ, Siewe R, Pongui B. Framing the peatlands governance in the Congo Basin. 2022. Available from: books.google.com

[55] Suzuki H, Masaoka T, Kurabayashi K, Ishii H, Kitajima M, Nomoto K, et al. Effect of dietary anti-urease immunoglobulin Y on *Helicobacter pylori* Infection in Mongolian Gerbils. Alimentary Pharmacology & Therapeutics. 2005

[56] Shahin AI, Zaib S, Zaraei SO, Kedia RA, Anbar HS. Design and synthesis of novel anti-urease imidazothiazole derivatives with promising antibacterial activity against *Helicobacter pylori*. PLoS One. 2023. Available from: journals.plos.org

[57] Mony TJ, Kwon HS, Won MK, Kang YM, Lee SH, Kim SY, et al. Anti-urease immunoglobulin (IgY) from egg yolk prevents *Helicobacter pylori* infection in a mouse model. Food and Agricultural Immunology. 2019

Section 2

Modern Treatment Modalities in Gastric Cancer

Chapter 4

Translating Molecular Subtypes into Clinical Practice: Precision Medicine in Gastric Cancer

Eunji Jang, Min-Kyue Shin, Jae-Ho Cheong and Yong-Min Huh

Abstract

Advancements in the handling of comprehensive genetic data in cancer research have led to the expansion of molecular subtyping studies. These studies reflect not only conventional tumor biological prognostic factors but also strive to develop predictive testing for therapeutic responses. While significant progress has been achieved, with commercial-grade assays now routinely used in breast cancer, similar efforts are currently underway in gastric cancer. In this review, we shed light on the current consensus in molecular subtyping research in gastric cancer and explore the potential of identified molecular signatures for the development of prognostic and predictive testing. Additionally, we address the unique characteristics of gastric cancer that present challenges for the straightforward development of successful prognostic/predictive tests. Drawing from these insights, we provide recommendations for incorporating prognostic testing into clinical treatment options and highlight key considerations for the successful advancement of predictive testing research.

Keywords: molecular subtyping, clinical decision making, precision medicine, prognostic test, predictive molecular marker

1. Introduction

Gastric cancer remains one of the most challenging malignancies to treat, with a high global incidence and mortality rate [1]. Despite advancements in surgical techniques and systemic therapies, the prognosis for patients with advanced gastric cancer is still poor [2]. This grim reality underscores the urgent need for a more personalized approach to treatment, one that can accurately predict therapeutic responses and improve patient outcomes [3].

Precision medicine, which tailors treatment based on the individual characteristics of each patient, has emerged as a promising strategy in this regard [4]. Central to this approach is the concept of molecular subtyping, a technique that classifies tumors based on their molecular and genetic profiles [5–7]. Molecular subtyping has revolutionized cancer treatment in several malignancies, most notably breast cancer, where it has led to the development of personalized therapies and improved survival rates [8, 9].

In gastric cancer, molecular subtyping studies have made significant strides, with several subtypes identified that reflect not only conventional tumor biological prognostic factors but also potential predictive markers for therapeutic responses [10, 11]. However, the translation of these findings into clinical practice has been challenging due to the unique characteristics of gastric cancer and the complexities involved in developing reliable prognostic and predictive tests [12, 13].

This review embarks on a recapitulative exploration of the current state of molecular subtyping in gastric cancer, emphasizing its ramifications for the burgeoning field of precision medicine. The ensuing chapters provide a detailed examination of the existing consensus within molecular subtyping research for gastric cancer, the insights gleaned from single-cell RNA sequencing, the potential integration of prognostic testing into clinical treatment modalities, and the key considerations that must be addressed to propel the successful advancement of predictive testing research.

By furnishing a comprehensive overview of the present landscape of molecular subtyping in gastric cancer and its prospective applications in precision medicine, this review aspires to contribute to the relentless efforts aimed at ameliorating the prognosis and treatment outcomes for patients afflicted with this devastating disease.

2. The current consensus in molecular subtyping research in gastric cancer

High-throughput gene expression profiling/sequencing technologies have opened new doors in understanding the molecular landscape of various cancers [14]. Molecular subtyping, which classifies tumors based on their molecular and genetic profiles, has become an essential tool in cancer research and in clinical practice. It sheds not only light on the biological behavior of tumors but also paves the way for personalized therapeutic strategies. In the field of gastric cancer, significant strides in molecular subtyping have been made by several research groups, including the Singapore group [15], The Cancer Genome Atlas (TCGA) [16], the Asian Cancer Research Group (ACRG) [17], the MD Anderson (MDACC) group [18], the Yonsei Cancer Center (YCC) [19], and the Mayo-Yonsei group [20].

In the early 2010s, the Singapore group identified three distinct molecular subtypes of gastric adenocarcinoma from 248 primary tumors: mesenchymal, proliferative, and metabolic subtypes [15]. The mesenchymal subtype was characterized by features of cancer stem cells, suggesting a more aggressive and undifferentiated state. The proliferative subtype was characterized by high levels of genomic instability, TP53 mutations, and DNA hypomethylation, indicative of a more chaotic genetic landscape. The metabolic subtype, on the other hand, was defined by gene sets related to metabolism pathways, reflecting a unique metabolic profile. While no significant survival difference was observed among the three subtypes ($P = 0.310$), the study revealed that the molecular subtypes may hold potential as they were associated with different sensitivities to chemotherapy drugs.

In 2014, TCGA provided a comprehensive molecular evaluation of 295 primary gastric adenocarcinomas, proposing a classification that divides gastric cancer into four distinct subtypes: Epstein–Barr virus (EBV) positive, microsatellite instability (MSI), genomically stable tumors (GS), and tumors with chromosomal instability (CIN) [16]. Each subtype has unique characteristics and implications for patient stratification and targeted therapies. Although these subtypes did not show a correlation with overall survival, Sohn et al. reported that they developed a TCGA subtype prediction model, showing that the EBV subtype was associated with the best prognosis and the GS subtype was associated with the worst prognosis in two independent retrospective cohorts ($P = 0.004$ and 0.03 in two cohorts, respectively). [20].

The ACRG analyzed 300 primary gastric adenocarcinomas, identifying four molecular subtypes: Microsatellite Stable with Epithelial-to-Mesenchymal Transition (MSS/EMT), Microsatellite Instability (MSI), TP53-active (MSS/TP53+), and TP53-inactive (MSS/TP53-) [17]. These subtypes are associated with unique genomic alterations, survival outcomes, and recurrence patterns. The MSS/EMT subtype, characterized by a mesenchymal-like type, has the worst prognosis and highest recurrence frequency, while the MSI subtype, linked to the hyper-mutated intestinal-subtype, has the best prognosis and lowest recurrence frequency. The study found statistically significant correlations with overall survival, with variations in outcomes and recurrence rates among the subtypes ($P < 0.001$, log-rank test for overall trend). These subtypes have potential implications for prognosis and treatment, with distinct characteristics and therapeutic strategies needed for each subtype.

The MDACC group identified two distinct molecular subtypes: mesenchymal phenotype (MP) and epithelial phenotype (EP) [18]. They revealed that the MP subtype is characterized by high genomic integrity, low mutation rates, EMT pathway, and microsatellite stability. Clinically, the MP subtype is associated with poor survival rates and resistance to standard chemotherapy, whereas the EP subtype is linked with better survival rates and sensitivity to chemotherapy.

The YCC study identified five biological subtypes of gastric cancer: Inflammatory (INF), Intestinal (INT), Gastric (GST), Intestinal with stemness (INT/S), and Mesenchymal (MSC) [19]. Each of these subtypes has distinct characteristics and implications for prognosis and treatment. The study found that the INF subtype showed a favorable prognosis while two of these subtypes, INT/S and MSC, had a dismal prognosis and expressed the Epithelial-to-Mesenchymal Transition (EMT) signature, indicating different molecular mechanisms driving the EMT phenotype in gastric cancer. The study also identified the Transforming Growth Factor-beta (TGF-β) pathway as a potential therapeutic target to reverse mesenchymal gene expression in both subtypes.

The Mayo-Yonsei study identified four molecular subtypes that are prognostic for survival and predictive of treatment response [20]. Specifically, Group 1 tumors overexpress genes related to the cell cycle and DNA repair, Group 2 lacks a distinct pattern, Group 3 tumors overexpress genes in apoptosis signaling and cell proliferation, and Group 4 tumors overexpress genes in TGF-β, SMAD, estrogen signaling, and mesenchymal morphogenesis pathways. The molecular subtypes are found to predict response to adjuvant 5-fluorouracil and platinum therapy after gastrectomy and to immune checkpoint inhibitors in patients with metastatic or recurrent disease.

A summary table for the five studies above is presented in **Table 1**. The five studies have each proposed different molecular subtypes of gastric cancer. While each classification system is unique, it is notable that the molecular subtypes identified through unsupervised learning often correlate with the cancer microenvironment, a connection that also has implications for prognosis. Despite variations in methodologies across the studies, a mesenchymal signature, stem-like feature, or the EMT signature, emerges as the most defining feature. This signature specifically isolates subtypes with poor prognosis (such as mesenchymal, GS, MSS/EMT, MP, MSC, and group 4) from other types of gastric cancer. Conversely, subtypes associated with a favorable prognosis, including EBV, MSI, and INF, are often linked to immune activity, particularly reflecting the function of cytotoxic T cells. This pattern linking molecular characteristics and prognosis was further observed independently: Zeng et al.

Studies	TCGA [16]	ACRG [17]	YCC [19]	MDACC [18]	Singapore [15]	Mayo-Yonsei [20]
Molecular subtypes	MSI: hypermutable phenotype, elevated mutation rates, including mutations in genes like MLH1, a favorable prognosis	MSI: associated with hypermutation, mutations in genes such as KRAS, PI3K-PTEN-mTOR pathway, ALK, and ARID1A, enrichment of PIK3CA H1047R mutations, a favorable prognosis	INF: high expression of immune genes (CXCL9, GBP5, and NKG7), KEGG pathways of Inflammatory response, Interferon-gamma response, a favorable prognosis			
	EBV: recurrent PIK3CA mutations, extreme DNA hypermethylation, and amplification of JAK2, CD274 (PD-L1), and PDCD1LG2 (PD-L2) CD8+ T cell infiltrate and IFN-γ immune signature, favorable prognosis	MSS/TP53+: Intact TP53 activity, associated with EBV infection, higher prevalence of mutations in APC, ARID1A, KRAS, PIK3CA, and SMAD4, intermediate risk				
	CIN: extensive somatic copy number alterations, amplifications of receptor tyrosine kinases, including ERBB2, EGFR, and MET, and is associated with intestinal histological type	MSS/TP53-: highest prevalence of TP53 mutations, with a low frequency of other mutations, recurrent focal amplifications in ERBB2, EGFR, CCNE1, CCND1, MDM2, ROBO2, GATA6, and MYC were common and significantly enriched	INT: high expression of intestinal epithelial differentiation and proliferative genes, KEGG pathways: G2M checkpoint, E2F targets, relatively favorable prognosis INT/S: heterogeneous transit-amplifying features, high expression of cell cycle and intestinal epithelial differentiation-related genes, as well as EMT-related genes (COL11A1 and CTHRC1) and Wnt signaling genes (NKD2 and DKK3)	EP: low genomic integrity, associated with better survival rates and sensitivity to chemotherapy, significantly higher somatic mutation rate compared to MP subtype, less common among diffuse histologic type, with lower non-tumor content	Proliferative: a high number of TP53 mutations, genomic instability, and DNA hypomethylation, strongly associated with Lauren intestinal type histology	Group1: associated with the cell cycle and DNA repair Group2: lacks a distinct pattern Group3: overexpress genes in apoptosis signaling and cell proliferation

Studies	TCGA [16]	ACRG [17]	YCC [19]	MDACC [18]	Singapore [15]	Mayo-Yonsei [20]
			GST: related to digestion, high expression of gastric-specific genes TFF1, TFF2, and GKN1, intermediate prognosis		Metabolic: "normal" gastric mucosa gene expression profile	
	GS: a lack of significant somatic copy number alterations, mutations in genes like CDH1 and RHOA, and is associated with diffuse histological type	MSS/EMT: lower number of mutation events, associated with the worst prognosis among the subtypes, diffuse-subtype tumors. Occurs at an earlier age, poor prognosis	MSC: high expression of myogenetic (MYLK and MYH11) and EMT (SFRP1 and TAGLN) genes, associated with the TGF-β signaling, the worst prognosis	MP: low mutation rates, MSI, and substantially lower copy number loss, poor survival and resistance to standard chemotherapy, highly activated signaling pathways driving EMT and IGF1/IGF1R pathway, high expression of MYH11, RICTOR, and CAV11, common among diffuse histologic type, with higher non-tumor content	Mesenchymal: rare TP53 mutations, decreased CDH1 expression, and increased undifferentiated cell markers, displays mostly Lauren diffuse type histology	Group 4: overexpressed genes found in TGF-β, SMAD, estrogen signaling, and mesenchymal morphogenesis pathways, diffuse-type histology and perineural invasion, the worst outcome
Subtyping method	unsupervised clustering on data from six molecular platforms (array-based somatic copy number analysis, whole-exome sequencing, array-based DNA methylation profiling, messengerRNAsequencing, microRNA (miRNA) sequencing and reverse-phase protein array (RPPA))	principal component analysis (PCA)	nonnegative matrix factorization	unsupervised hierarchical clustering	consensus hierarchical clustering with iterative feature selection	NTriPath genetic signatures-based consensus clustering

Studies	TCGA [16]	ACRG [17]	YCC [19]	MDACC [18]	Singapore [15]	Mayo-Yonsei [20]
Training cohort	n = 295, Race White (59%), Asian (26%), Black or African-American (2%), Age median 68 (IQR 59–74), Sex male (62%), female (38%), Stage I (12%), II (40%), III (36%), IV (6%), Lauren intestinal (65%), diffuse (25%)	n = 300, Race Asian, Age median 64 (IQR 55–70), Sex male (66%), female (34%), Stage I (10%), II (32%), III (32%), IV (26%), Lauren intestinal (49%), diffuse (45%)	n = 547, Race Asian, Age median 61 (IQR 53–68), Sex male (68%), female (32%), Stage I (9%), II (28%), III (52%), IV (11%), Lauren intestinal (36%), diffuse (34%)	n = 93, Race Asian, Age median 60 (IQR 50–69), Sex male (78%), female (22%), Stage I (12%), II (19%), III (29%), IV (39%), Lauren intestinal (63%), diffuse (33%)	n = 248, Race Asian, Age median 67 (IQR 57–73), Sex male (65%), female (35%), Stage I (16%), II (15%), III (38%), IV (32%), Lauren intestinal (52%), diffuse (39%)	n = 567 Race Asian, Age less than 60 (48.5%), more than 60 (51.5%), Sex male (68.1%), female (31.9%), Stage I (3.7%), II (25.9%), III (66.8%), IV (3.5%), Lauren intestinal (34.2%), diffuse (34.9%)
Validation cohort	ACRG (GSE66229, n = 300), MDACC (GSE13861, GSE26899, and GSE26901, n = 267), SMC (GSE26253, n = 432)	SMC-2 (GSE26253, n = 277), Singapore cohort (GSE15459, n = 200), TCGA-STAD (n = 205)	Singapore cohort (GSE15459, n = 200), ACRG (GSE66229, n = 300)	YUSH (GSE13861, n = 65), KUCM (GSE26901, n = 109), SMC (GSE26253, n = 432), ACRG (GSE66229, n = 300), MDACC (GSE28541, n = 40)	Australian cohort (n = 70)	TCGA-STAD (n = 205), ACRG (GSE66229, n = 300), Sohn et al. cohort (GSE13861 and GSE26942, n = 267)

Table 1.
A summary table for the five studies of molecular subtypes in gastric cancer.

proposed TMEclusters that were associated with prognosis [21]. They identified these clusters through computational analysis that inferred infiltrating cell types within the tumor microenvironment. Specifically, TMEcluster-A, marked by high infiltration of cancer-associated fibroblasts, M2 macrophages, resting dendritic cells, and resting mast cells, was associated with a poor prognosis. Conversely, TMEcluster-C, characterized by a significant increase in the infiltration of CD8+ T cells, M1 macrophages, and activated memory CD4+ T cells, was linked to a favorable prognosis.

While there is a growing consensus on molecular subtypes influenced by the cancer microenvironment, the intrinsic molecular subtypes specific to gastric cancer remain relatively less explored. The Singapore group identified not only mesenchymal types but also proliferative and metabolic subtypes. In contrast, the TCGA pinpointed CIN types alongside EBV, MSI, and GS subtypes. The ACRG's classification incorporated TP53 activation, in addition to MSI and EMT types, while the MDACC group identified EP types as a counterpart of MP type. The YCC study differentiated between gastric and intestinal types.

When examining gene signature expression, similarities emerge. For instance, both the metabolic subtype from the Singapore group and the gastric type from the YCC study exhibit gene signatures associated with digestion. The intestinal type, on the other hand, displays gene expression patterns linked to not only features of the intestinal epithelium but also proliferation for the cell cycle. It is noteworthy that tumor-infiltrating T cells also exhibit proliferative gene expression when compared to peripheral blood mononuclear cells [22]. This suggests that in the Singapore group's molecular subtype classification, which does not differentiate immune-active molecular subtypes, the proliferative group might represent a blend of both intestinal and inflammatory types. However, the situation becomes more complex when considering the TP53 activation-driven subtype identified by the ACRG and the CIN subtype defined by the TCGA. Since neither of these subtypes has been characterized by specific gene signature expression, it becomes challenging to draw direct comparisons or establish correlations with the subtypes identified by the Singapore group or the YCC. In the YCC study, the majority of INT/S and GST type was identified as the TCGA CIN type. The INT type was further categorized into MSI and CIN in the TCGA subtypes, suggesting the presence of an MSI subtype with reduced immune activity, compared to the INF type with MSI. Groups 1,2, and 3 from the Mayo-Yonsei group did not show direct correlations to the other subtypes.

Despite attempts to understand the consensus in the molecular subtypes in gastric cancer, the lack of defined gene signatures adds a layer of complexity to the task of integrating and reconciling these various subtype classifications, underscoring the need for further research to elucidate the underlying molecular characteristics.

3. Navigating cellular complexity: Single-cell RNA-seq in gastric cancer research

Molecular subtyping through bulk RNA-seq has significantly advanced our understanding of the heterogeneity in gastric cancer [15–19]. However, the inherent limitations of bulk RNA-seq, especially its low resolution, constrain the ability to discern variability and interactions among cancer cells when they are mixed with different cell types, such as immune and stromal cells [23]. While various deconvolution computational methods have been developed to infer cell type proportions from transcriptomic data, these results can be inconsistent, depending on factors like data conversion, preprocessing, marker selection, cell type composition, and the methodology employed [24, 25]. These challenges highlight the need for more precise techniques, leading to the development and adoption of single-cell RNA-seq methods [23, 26]. Unlike traditional approaches, single-cell sequencing offers a direct window into the cellular landscape, providing a more detailed and subtle view.

Building on the advancements in single-cell RNA sequencing, Sathe et al. examined 56,167 cells from seven gastric cancer (GC) patients, one patient with intestinal metaplasia, paired normal tissue, and peripheral blood mononuclear cells, revealing substantial heterogeneity within both the tumor epithelium [27]. Their study identified three distinct subclasses of epithelial cells: GC type 1, GC type 2, and normal gastric epithelial cells. The GC type 1 subclass was characterized by increased expression of intestinal mucosa markers, while the GC type 2 subclass exhibited a significant upregulation of known gastric cancer marker genes. These findings underscore the ability of single-cell RNA sequencing to provide detailed insights into the complex cellular landscape of gastric cancer, allowing for a more nuanced understanding of the disease at the individual cell level.

A pivotal example of this advancement is the study conducted by Zhang et al., where they performed single-cell RNA sequencing on 27,677 cells from 9 tumors and 3 non-tumor gastric adenocarcinoma samples [28]. Their comprehensive analysis identified five distinct cell subgroups (C1 ~ C5), uncovering the intricate transcriptional landscape heterogeneity within gastric adenocarcinoma malignant cells. Notably, the samples corresponding to the Lauren intestinal type were further divided into four distinct subgroups (C2 to C5), each displaying varying degrees of differentiation. Moreover, the study's approach led to the identification of a rare variant of gastric cancer (C4) and revealed a more cycling lymphoid cell population (in the S and G2M phases) in the intestinal-type EBV-positive patient (C5).

Another recent study by Kim et al. analyzed 30,888 cells from 24 GC patients, identifying eight sub-cell populations within 1003 tumor cells, with specific markers for intestinal gastric cancer (IGC) and diffuse gastric cancer (DGC) being highly expressed in different clusters [29]. All the sub-cell populations were categorized into ACRG subtypes, particularly EMT (C0, C3, C4, C6, and C7). Interestingly, the C5 group did not express EMT signatures but were enriched in markers of the epithelial–myofibroblast transition (EmyoT), significantly correlated with poor overall survival, followed by the EMT. This discovery highlights that, although cancer-associated fibroblasts are frequently attributed to the mesenchymal or EMT feature in bulk RNA-seq transcriptome analyses, the sub-populations within isolated tumor cells can be distinctly characterized by EMT and EmyoT signatures, revealing a more nuanced understanding of their roles and behaviors.

The studies utilizing scRNA-seq have shed light on the complex heterogeneity within gastric cancer cells and the various cell populations in the gastric cancer microenvironment. For instance, Kumar et al.'s recent work created an extensive single-cell atlas of gastric cancer by analyzing over 200,000 cells from 29 samples across 31 patients, identifying 34 unique cell-lineage states [30]. This included rare cell populations in transition and specific expression programs for different cell types, revealing that a higher presence of plasma cells was associated with KLF2 expression diffuse-type gastric cancers and that a unique fibroblast type with high co-expression of INHBA and FAP was linked to a lower overall survival rate. Other researchers, such as Fu et al. explored the immune landscape, describing various immune cell subtypes and tracing their developmental paths [31]. They identified the downregulation of the IRF8 transcription factor in CD8+ tumor-infiltrating lymphocytes and its association with more advanced disease stages in gastric cancer patients, offering a basis for targeted immune therapy. Eum et al. constructed a reference macrophage transcriptome at the single-cell level, finding noninflammatory characteristics in macrophages and M2-specific signatures associated with poor prognosis [32]. Kim et al. discerned three CAF types, inflammatory (iCAF), myofibroblastic (myCAF), and intermediate CAFs (inCAF), based on gene expression states [29]. In their findings, iCAFs, more prevalent in diffuse-type gastric cancers, are linked to invasion and tumor cell stemness, while myCAFs are more common in intestinal-type gastric cancers, emphasizing the complex roles of CAFs and their potential influence on tumor structures and interactions within the tumor microenvironment. In addition, scRNA-seq also reveals information about the arrangement of epithelial cells near the cancer site. Zhang et al. built a single-cell network for epithelial cells in early gastric cancer and premalignant lesions, characterizing cell transitions in metaplasia and in the early-malignant lesion [33]. Collectively, these advancements lay the groundwork for the development of more personalized, targeted, and effective therapeutic strategies for gastric cancer in the future.

4. From gastric cancer heterogeneity: incorporating prognostic testing into clinical treatment options

While systematic studies based on the high-throughput gene profiling and sequencing data are currently being conducted across various types of cancer, it was within the specialized domain of breast cancer that these scientific endeavors first realized the successful commercialization of prognostic and predictive tests at the clinical level [34, 35]. In the early 2000s, while unsupervised learning methodologies were applied to explore heterogeneity within the transcriptome [14], prognostic tests were concurrently developed using supervised approaches, complemented by the integration of clinical information [36, 37]. These efforts developed prognostic assays, such as Oncotype Dx and Mammaprint, which provide personalized information about the likelihood of cancer recurrence and the potential benefit of chemotherapy for women with early-stage, hormone-receptor-positive breast cancer. Further scholarly exploration has uncovered the role of proliferative gene expression as a determinant axis for prognostication [38]. The clinical efficacy of these assays has been thoroughly corroborated through extensive clinical trials and has been integrated into esteemed treatment protocols, including those endorsed by the National Comprehensive Cancer Network (NCCN) and the American Society of Clinical Oncology (ASCO) [39–41].

The achievement of commercializing prognostic and predictive tests in breast cancer may appear as a straightforward benchmark; however, the unique tumor biology of gastric cancer presents formidable challenges to such benchmarking. In 2011, Cho et al. devised a six-gene-based risk scoring system, employing unsupervised clustering and Cox hazard scoring on transcriptomic data [42]. Despite its prognostic performance, the collective biological attributes represented by the six genes remained unidentified. Subsequently, in 2013, Wu et al. conducted a comprehensive meta-analysis of transcriptomic data, revealing that the expression of a stroma-related "super-module" was intricately associated with transforming growth factor beta (TGF-β) signaling and the stromal-related expression consistently served as a prognostic indicator across multiple gastric cancer cohorts [43]. Park et al. identified ACTA2 as a prognostic marker for gastric cancer using previous studies [19, 20] and validated using pooled data from 3 large independent cohorts [44]. Parallel molecular subtype studies have consistently observed that the expression of stromal features (mesenchymal, stem-like, or EMT) portends a poor prognosis, a finding that stands different from observations in breast cancer. In gastric cancer, the presence of stromal features was concomitant with reduced proliferative gene expression, and it appeared that patients exhibiting the stromal feature gained minimal therapeutic benefit from adjuvant cancer treatment [15, 17–21, 45]. Meanwhile, gastric cancer molecular subtyping studies have identified distinct groups characterized by immune activity, including EBV, MSI, and INF subtypes [16, 17, 19, 21, 45]. These patient categories have been independently associated with favorable prognoses. Immunohistochemistry-based investigations have further corroborated that the infiltration of cytotoxic T cells within cancerous tissues is concomitant with a favorable prognosis and a diminished likelihood of benefiting from chemotherapy [46].

In light of the specific observations, Cheong and colleagues engineered the Single Patient Classifier (SPC), comprising immune (IM), stem-like (ST), and epithelial (EP) classifiers [47]. Their study was designed with the objective of formulating and validating a predictive examination for the prognosis and the response to adjuvant chemotherapy in patients with resectable, stage II–III gastric cancer. Within the validation cohort exploiting the CLASSIC trial archived samples, this prognostic SPC discerned disparate risk categories, independently of the TNM system, while the predictive SPC allocated patients into groups characterized by either a benefit or a lack of benefit from chemotherapy.

In contrast to the breast cancer testing, SPC testing in gastric cancer is distinguished by a bifurcated structure, segregating prognostic and predictive SPC. While the prognostic SPC encompasses IM and ST classifiers, the predictive SPC isolates patients with high EP expression from a subgroup that omits IM-high patients with favorable prognosis. Rather than the SPC employing a binary division to categorize patients into EP and ST subtypes, the algorithm permits nuanced distinctions within the ST and EP classifiers, such as the identification of patients who are double positive for ST and EP classifiers. This algorithm design was intended according to the observation of a specific subset of INT/S (intestinal type with stem-like feature) within transcriptomic molecular subtyping studies. Precisely, among patients who evade classification as stromal type (MP, EMT, or ST) due to the pronounced overexpression of epithelial signature genes, there exists a cohort that manifests expression of stem-like or EMT genes, whose prognosis aligns with the poor outcomes typically associated with the stromal type [19, 47]. Further investigation will be required to understand the cellular-level heterogeneity observed in these patients.

Currently, in South Korea, additional prospective multicenter clinical trials are being conducted to validate the performance of the SPC test. A retrospective trial encompassing approximately 2000 cases has recently reached completion. Within the clinical community, deliberations are underway to explore avenues for integrating SPC results into the prevailing TNM staging system-based treatment paradigms. For instance, informed by the SPC test results, physicians may advocate for more aggressive chemotherapy protocols for individuals classified within the high-risk category in stage II. Conversely, they may elect to forego chemotherapy or opt for milder regimens for those identified as low-risk within stages II and III. Such determinations must be judiciously rendered, with paramount consideration given to patient safety [13, 48]. The formulation of SPC-based treatment guidelines may necessitate the initiation of supplementary clinical trials. Concurrently, building on antecedent research wherein the SPC risk group was substantiated as an independent prognostic factor relative to the conventional TNM staging system, currently the most powerful tool for prognostication, Choi et al. have advanced a modified TNM staging proposal [49]. This approach incorporates SPC information through a one-grade down-staging for patients delineated within the low-risk group, culminating in an enhancement of the C-index. It merits acknowledgment that the SPC test, originally devised for advanced gastric cancer, has been cited in reports as having the capacity to discern a specific subgroup of patients who are at an elevated risk even in the context of early gastric cancer [50, 51].

5. Key considerations for the successful advancement of predictive testing research

Current treatment protocols for gastric cancer primarily rely on TNM staging, which guides postoperative monitoring for early-stage cases, adjuvant cancer therapy for advanced stages, and palliative care for late-stage conditions [52, 53]. Nonetheless, varying stages of the disease exhibit different responses to treatments, highlighting the necessity for predictive markers to tailor therapeutic approaches.

In response to this unmet clinical need, the predictive efficacy of treatment response was assessed based on molecular subtypes in gastric cancer. Sohn et al. reported that the TCGA CIN subtype had the benefit from adjuvant chemotherapy (HR, 0.39; 95% CI, 0.16–0.94; P = 0.03) and those with the GS subtype had the least benefit from adjuvant chemotherapy (HR, 0.83; 95% CI, 0.36–1.89; P = 0.65) [45]. The MDACC group revealed that the EP subtype was associated with a favorable response to chemotherapy (HR 0.42 95% CI 0.22–0.8, P = 0.004 by likelihood ratio test) while the MP subtype demonstrated resistance to standard chemotherapy (P = 0.98 by likelihood ratio test) [18]. The Mayo-Yonsei study disclosed that Group 3 showed a favorable response to treatment with 5-FU plus platinum (HR 0.28, 95% CI 0.08–0.96, P = 0.043). In contrast, treatment did not significantly impact survival outcomes for patients in Groups 2 and 4. For Group 1, those who were administered 5-FU plus platinum experienced poorer survival compared to those who did not undergo adjuvant therapy, with an HR of 6.80 (95% CI, 1.46–31.6, P = 0.015) [20]. While these findings are intriguing, they lack robust evidence due to limitations such as retrospective data collection and inadequate sample size. To improve the evidence level, the predictive efficacy of the SPC was assessed using archived specimens from the CLASSIC trial (a multicentered, randomized, open-label, and phase 3 trial), in accordance with the principle of "prospective–retrospective designs for evaluating prognostic and predictive biomarkers," as outlined by Simon et al. [54]. In the group predicted to benefit from chemotherapy, the 5-year overall survival rate was notably higher for patients who underwent adjuvant chemotherapy post-surgery compared to those who only had surgery (univariate HR 0.47 [95% CI 0.30–0.75], p = 0.0015). Conversely, no such increase in 5-year overall survival was seen in the group predicted to not benefit from chemotherapy (univariate HR 0.93 [0.62–1.38], p = 0.71) [47].

Immune checkpoint inhibitors (ICIs) have become not only the standard of treatment in stage IV gastric cancer but also could be further approved in the perioperative setting, considering a promising result from the interim analysis of the phase 3 MATTERHORN trial (NCT04592913) [55]. However, there was no survival benefit from both nivolumab and pembrolizumab in patients with low programmed death-ligand 1 (PD-L1) expression [56]. On the contrary, microsatellite instability-high (MSI-H) patients exhibited outstanding benefits from pembrolizumab, regardless of the line of ICI therapy [57]. Tumor mutational burden (TMB) was also a significant predictive biomarker for the ICI response, although its utility was attenuated after the exclusion of MSI-H patients [58, 59]. In addition, patients with EBV-positive tumors showed a remarkable response to pembrolizumab monotherapy in a phase 2 trial [60], in line with the association of EBV with PD-L1 overexpression and immune cell signaling [16]. Assessment of these biomarkers is useful not only in the palliative setting but also could be used as biomarkers in patients with operable gastric cancer. Specifically, MSI-H and PD-L1 expression in stromal immune cells were associated with favorable prognosis and non-responsiveness to perioperative chemotherapy in post hoc analyses of two phase 3 trials [61, 62]. Furthermore, the associations between gene expression signatures and response to medical treatments have been demonstrated recently. In an exploratory analysis from the KEYNOTE-061 trial, T-cell-inflamed gene expression profile was associated with a good response to pembrolizumab, while monocytic myeloid-derived suppressor cell signature was associated with a poor response to pembrolizumab [63]. In another study, TGF-β signaling genes were associated with non-responsiveness to both adjuvant chemotherapy and palliative ICI therapies [20]. Additionally, expression of a single gene, ACTA2, was negatively associated with response to ICIs in a study of multiple cohorts [44]. A comprehensive examination of the aforementioned molecular markers will be helpful for the appropriate selection of treatment strategies.

Recent positive results from clinical trials of targeted agents will likely further change treatment standards for gastric cancer. In the phase 3 SPOTLIGHT trial, which included untreated patients with claudin-18 isoform 2 (CLDN18.2) positive stage IV gastric cancer, the combination of zolbetuximab with chemotherapy significantly reduced the risk of disease progression or death with a hazard ratio (HR) of 0.75 [64]. In the phase 3 GLOW trial, which was almost the same as the SPOTLIGHT study except for the conventional chemotherapy regimen, the addition of zolbetuximab significantly prolonged progression-free survival (PFS) (HR = 0.69) and overall survival (OS) (HR = 0.77) [65]. High expression of CLDN18.2 in gastric cancer with diffuse, undifferentiated, and signet ring cell histology [66–68], which are associated with poor prognosis and non-responsiveness to ICIs, makes it an even more appealing therapeutic target, although CLDN18.2 expression itself was not associated with prognosis nor ICI response in a retrospective single-institution study [69]. In addition, the phase 2 FIGHT trial demonstrated promising efficacy (HR = 0.68 for PFS and HR = 0.60 for OS) of bemarituzumab, a fibroblast growth factor receptor 2 isoform IIb (FGFR2b)-targeting agent [70], and the phase 3 FORTITUDE-101 trial is ongoing. Given that FGFR2 amplification is associated with poor prognosis in gastric cancer [71], its therapeutic targeting will be of great clinical benefit.

Numerous translational studies have presented novel therapeutic opportunities for the SEM (Stem-like/Epithelial-to-mesenchymal transition/Mesenchymal) subtype gastric cancer. Intrinsic tumor expression and dependency of TGF-β signaling were demonstrated in clinical samples and preclinical models of the mesenchymal subtype gastric cancer [19]. Furthermore, erythrocyte membrane protein band 4.1-like 5 (EPB41L5) was identified as a mediator of TGF-β signaling-induced metastasis and its inhibition showed preclinical efficacy [72]. Synaptotagmin 11 was also identified as a therapeutic target of gastric cancer with the SEM subtype through transcriptomic analysis, mechanistic studies, and preclinical experiments [73]. Interestingly, several studies have discovered metabolic vulnerabilities of the SEM subtype gastric cancer. An inhibitor of nicotinamide phosphoribosyltransferase demonstrated selective toxicity against gastric cancer with the EMT subtype, due to its loss of nicotinic acid phosphoribosyltransferase [74]. Moreover, inhibition of plasma membrane calcium

ATPase reversed drug resistance in gastric cancer models derived from metabolic stress conditions [75]. In addition, glutaminase and phosphoglycerate dehydrogenase caused metabolic plasticity in the SEM subtype gastric cancer, which could be therapeutically exploited [76]. The polyunsaturated fatty acid biosynthesis pathway and ferroptosis were recognized as promising markers for treating mesenchymal-type gastric cancer in preclinical experiments [77].

6. Conclusion

The comprehensive examination of molecular subtyping in gastric cancer, as presented in this review, underscores its transformative potential in the field of oncology. Through the integration of high-throughput gene profiling, sequencing technologies, and single-cell RNA sequencing, a nuanced understanding of the molecular landscape of gastric cancer has been achieved. This understanding has paved the way for the identification of distinct subtypes, each with unique prognostic factors and therapeutic response markers. However, the translation of these scientific discoveries into clinical practice remains a complex endeavor, filled with challenges unique to the heterogeneous nature of gastric cancer. The insights gleaned from various research groups, including the Singapore group, TCGA, ACRG, MDACC, YCC, and Mayo-Yonsei have illuminated the path forward, yet the integration of these findings into a unified, actionable framework requires further exploration and validation.

As we approach a new phase in treating gastric cancer, the potential of personalized medicine becomes increasingly significant. The development and validation of prognostic and predictive tests, such as the SPC, signal a future where treatment can be tailored to the individual characteristics of each patient. The ongoing efforts in South Korea and other research centers worldwide to validate and incorporate these tests into existing treatment paradigms signify a concrete step toward this future. Yet, the journey is far from complete. Continued collaboration across research groups, rigorous clinical trials, and a steadfast commitment to patient safety and ethical considerations will be paramount in realizing the full potential of molecular subtyping in gastric cancer. The path is complex, but the potential rewards for patients and the broader medical community are profound. The pursuit of a more personalized, targeted, and effective therapeutic strategy for gastric cancer is not just a scientific aspiration; it is a moral imperative that holds the promise of transforming lives and redefining the future of cancer treatment.

Conflict of interest

J-HC and Y-MH are founders and shareholders of NOVOMICS. Other authors declare no competing interests.

Author details

Eunji Jang[1], Min-Kyue Shin[2], Jae-Ho Cheong[3,4,6,8,9]* and Yong-Min Huh[3,5,7,8,9]*

1 MediBio-Informatics Research Center, Novomics Co., Ltd., Seoul, Republic of Korea

2 Samsung Advanced Institute of Health Science and Technology, Sungkyunkwan University, Seoul, Republic of Korea

3 College of Medicine, Yonsei University, Seoul, Republic of Korea

4 Department of Surgery, Yonsei University, Seoul, Republic of Korea

5 Department of Radiology, Yonsei University, Seoul, Republic of Korea

6 Department of Biomedical Systems Informatics, Yonsei University, Seoul, Republic of Korea

7 YUHS-KRIBB Medical Convergence Research Institute, Seoul, Republic of Korea

8 Department of Biochemistry and Molecular Biology, College of Medicine, Yonsei University, Seoul, Republic of Korea

9 Brain Korea 21 Project for Medical Science, Yonsei University College of Medicine, Seoul, Republic of Korea

*Address all correspondence to: jhcheong@yuhs.ac; ymhuh@yuhs.ac

References

[1] Sung H, Ferlay J, Siegel RL, Laversanne M, Soerjomataram I, Jemal A, et al. Global cancer statistics 2020: GLOBOCAN estimates of incidence and mortality worldwide for 36 cancers in 185 countries. CA: A Cancer Journal for Clinicians. 2021;**71**(3):209-249. DOI: 10.3322/caac.21660

[2] Li Y, Feng A, Zheng S, Chen C, Lyu J. Recent estimates and predictions of 5-year survival in patients with gastric cancer: A model-based period analysis. Cancer Control. 2022;**Jan29**:10732748221099227. DOI: 10.1177/10732748221099227

[3] Ajani JA, Lee J, Sano T, Janjigian YY, Fan D, Song S. Gastric adenocarcinoma. Natural Review Disease Primers. 2017;**3**:17036. DOI: 10.1038/nrdp.2017.36

[4] Tsimberidou AM, Fountzilas E, Nikanjam M, Kurzrock R. Review of precision cancer medicine: Evolution of the treatment paradigm. Cancer Treatment Reviews. 2020;**86**:102019. DOI: 10.1016/j.ctrv.2020.102019

[5] Grossman RL, Heath AP, Ferretti V, Varmus HE, Lowy DR, Kibbe WA, et al. Toward a shared vision for cancer genomic data. The New England Journal of Medicine. 2016;**375**(12):1109-1112. DOI: 10.1056/NEJMp1607591

[6] Dai X, Xiang L, Li T, Bai Z. Cancer hallmarks, biomarkers and breast Cancer molecular subtypes. Journal of Cancer. 2016;**7**(10):1281-1294. DOI: 10.7150/jca.13141

[7] Dienstmann R, Vermeulen L, Guinney J, Kopetz S, Tejpar S, Tabernero J. Consensus molecular subtypes and the evolution of precision medicine in colorectal cancer. Nature Reviews. Cancer. 2017;**17**(2):79-92. DOI: 10.1038/nrc.2016.126

[8] Paik S, Tang G, Shak S, Kim C, Baker J, Kim W, et al. Gene expression and benefit of chemotherapy in women with node-negative, estrogen receptor-positive breast cancer. Journal of Clinical Oncology. 2006;**24**(23):3726-3734. DOI: 10.1200/JCO.2005.04.7985

[9] Bang YJ, Van Cutsem E, Feyereislova A, Chung HC, Shen L, Sawaki A, et al. ToGA trial investigators. Trastuzumab in combination with chemotherapy versus chemotherapy alone for treatment of HER2-positive advanced gastric or gastro-oesophageal junction cancer (ToGA): A phase 3, open-label, randomised controlled trial. Lancet. 2010;**376**(9742):687-697. DOI: 10.1016/S0140-6736(10)61121-X

[10] Zeng Y, Jin RU. Molecular pathogenesis, targeted therapies, and future perspectives for gastric cancer. Seminars in Cancer Biology. 2022;**86**(Pt 3):566-582. DOI: 10.1016/j.semcancer.2021.12.004

[11] Niclauss N, Gütgemann I, Dohmen J, Kalff JC, Lingohr P. Novel biomarkers of gastric adenocarcinoma: Current research and future perspectives. Cancers (Basel). 2021;**13**(22):5660. DOI: 10.3390/cancers13225660

[12] Riley RD, Sauerbrei W, Altman DG. Prognostic markers in cancer: The evolution of evidence from single studies to meta-analysis, and beyond. British Journal of Cancer. 2009;**100**(8):1219-1229. DOI: 10.1038/sj.bjc.6604999

[13] Boracchi P, Biganzoli E. Markers of prognosis and response to treatment: Ready for clinical use in oncology?

A biostatistician's viewpoint. The International Journal of Biological Markers. 2003;**18**(1):65-69. DOI: 10.1177/172460080301800112

[14] Perou CM, Sørlie T, Eisen MB, van de Rijn M, Jeffrey SS, Rees CA, et al. Molecular portraits of human breast tumours. Nature. 2000;**406**(6797):747-752. DOI: 10.1038/35021093

[15] Lei Z, Tan IB, Das K, Deng N, Zouridis H, Pattison S, et al. Identification of molecular subtypes of gastric cancer with different responses to PI3-kinase inhibitors and 5-fluorouracil. Gastroenterology. 2013;**145**(3):554-565. DOI: 10.1053/j.gastro.2013.05.010

[16] Cancer Genome Atlas Research Network. Comprehensive molecular characterization of gastric adenocarcinoma. Nature. 2014;**513**(7517):202-209. DOI: 10.1038/nature13480

[17] Cristescu R, Lee J, Nebozhyn M, Kim KM, Ting JC, Wong SS, et al. Molecular analysis of gastric cancer identifies subtypes associated with distinct clinical outcomes. Nature Medicine. 2015;**21**(5):449-456. DOI: 10.1038/nm.3850

[18] Oh SC, Sohn BH, Cheong JH, Kim SB, Lee JE, Park KC, et al. Clinical and genomic landscape of gastric cancer with a mesenchymal phenotype. Nature Communications. 2018;**9**(1):1777. DOI: 10.1038/s41467-018-04179-8

[19] Jang E, Shin MK, Kim H, Lim JY, Lee JE, Park J, et al. Clinical molecular subtyping reveals intrinsic mesenchymal reprogramming in gastric cancer cells. Experimental & Molecular Medicine. 2023;**55**(5):974-986. DOI: 10.1038/s12276-023-00989-z

[20] Cheong JH, Wang SC, Park S, Porembka MR, Christie AL, Kim H, et al. Development and validation of a prognostic and predictive 32-gene signature for gastric cancer. Nature Communications. 2022;**13**(1):774. DOI: 10.1038/s41467-022-28437-y

[21] Zeng D, Li M, Zhou R, Zhang J, Sun H, Shi M, et al. Tumor microenvironment characterization in gastric cancer identifies prognostic and Immunotherapeutically relevant gene signatures. Cancer Immunology Research. 2019;7(5):737-750. DOI: 10.1158/2326-6066.CIR-18-0436

[22] Yang B, Chou J, Tao Y, Wu D, Wu X, Li X, et al. An assessment of prognostic immunity markers in breast cancer. NPJ Breast Cancer. 2018;**4**:35. DOI: 10.1038/s41523-018-0088-0

[23] Fan J, Slowikowski K, Zhang F. Single-cell transcriptomics in cancer: Computational challenges and opportunities. Experimental & Molecular Medicine. 2020;**52**(9):1452-1465. DOI: 10.1038/s12276-020-0422-0

[24] Chen B, Khodadoust MS, Liu CL, Newman AM, Alizadeh AA. Profiling tumor infiltrating immune cells with CIBERSORT. Methods in Molecular Biology. 2018;**1711**:243-259. DOI: 10.1007/978-1-4939-7493-1_12

[25] Avila Cobos F, Alquicira-Hernandez J, Powell JE, Mestdagh P, De Preter K. Benchmarking of cell type deconvolution pipelines for transcriptomics data. Nature Communications. 2020;**11**(1):5650. DOI: 10.1038/s41467-020-19015-1

[26] Zhang Y, Wang D, Peng M, Tang L, Ouyang J, Xiong F, et al. Single-cell RNA sequencing in cancer research. Journal of Experimental & Clinical Cancer Research. 2021;**40**(1):81. DOI: 10.1186/s13046-021-01874-1

[27] Sathe A, Grimes SM, Lau BT, Chen J, Suarez C, Huang RJ, et al. Single-cell

genomic characterization reveals the cellular reprogramming of the gastric tumor microenvironment. Clinical Cancer Research. 2020;**26**(11):2640-2653. DOI: 10.1158/1078-0432.CCR-19-3231

[28] Zhang M, Hu S, Min M, Ni Y, Lu Z, Sun X, et al. Dissecting transcriptional heterogeneity in primary gastric adenocarcinoma by single cell RNA sequencing. Gut. 2021;**70**(3):464-475. DOI: 10.1136/gutjnl-2019-320368

[29] Kim J, Park C, Kim KH, Kim EH, Kim H, Woo JK, et al. Single-cell analysis of gastric pre-cancerous and cancer lesions reveals cell lineage diversity and intratumoral heterogeneity. NPJ Precision Oncology. 2022;**6**(1):9. DOI: 10.1038/s41698-022-00251-1

[30] Kumar V, Ramnarayanan K, Sundar R, Padmanabhan N, Srivastava S, Koiwa M, et al. Single-cell atlas of lineage states, tumor microenvironment, and subtype-specific expression programs in gastric cancer. Cancer Discovery. 2022;**12**(3):670-691. DOI: 10.1158/2159-8290.CD-21-0683

[31] Fu K, Hui B, Wang Q, Lu C, Shi W, Zhang Z, et al. Single-cell RNA sequencing of immune cells in gastric cancer patients. Aging (Albany NY). 2020;**12**(3):2747-2763. DOI: 10.18632/aging.102774

[32] Eum HH, Kwon M, Ryu D, Jo A, Chung W, Kim N, et al. Tumor-promoting macrophages prevail in malignant ascites of advanced gastric cancer. Experimental & Molecular Medicine. 2020;**52**(12):1976-1988. DOI: 10.1038/s12276-020-00538-y

[33] Zhang P, Yang M, Zhang Y, Xiao S, Lai X, Tan A, et al. Dissecting the single-cell transcriptome network underlying gastric premalignant lesions and early gastric cancer. Cell Reports. 2019;**27**(6):1934-1947.e5. DOI: 10.1016/j.celrep.2019.04.052

[34] Győrffy B, Hatzis C, Sanft T, Hofstatter E, Aktas B, Pusztai L. Multigene prognostic tests in breast cancer: Past, present, future. Breast Cancer Research. 2015;**17**(1):11. DOI: 10.1186/s13058-015-0514-2

[35] Goossens N, Nakagawa S, Sun X, Hoshida Y. Cancer biomarker discovery and validation. Translational Cancer Research. 2015;**4**(3):256-269. DOI: 10.3978/j.issn.2218-676X.2015.06.04

[36] van de Vijver MJ, He YD, et al. A gene-expression signature as a predictor of survival in breast cancer. The New England Journal of Medicine. 2002;**347**(25):1999-2009. DOI: 10.1056/NEJMoa021967

[37] Paik S, Shak S, Tang G, Kim C, Baker J, Cronin M, et al. A multigene assay to predict recurrence of tamoxifen-treated, node-negative breast cancer. The New England Journal of Medicine. 2004;**351**(27):2817-2826. DOI: 10.1056/NEJMoa041588

[38] Wirapati P, Sotiriou C, Kunkel S, Farmer P, Pradervand S, Haibe-Kains B, et al. Meta-analysis of gene expression profiles in breast cancer: Toward a unified understanding of breast cancer subtyping and prognosis signatures. Breast Cancer Research. 2008;**10**(4):R65. DOI: 10.1186/bcr2124

[39] Sparano JA, Gray RJ, Makower DF, Pritchard KI, Albain KS, Hayes DF, et al. Adjuvant chemotherapy guided by a 21-gene expression assay in breast cancer. The New England Journal of Medicine. 2018;**379**(2):111-121. DOI: 10.1056/NEJMoa1804710

[40] National Comprehensive Cancer Network. Clinical Practice Guidelines in

Oncology. Breast Cancer. Version 4. 2023. Available from: https://www.nccn.org/professionals/physician_gls/pdf/breast.pdf [Accessed: August 27, 2023]

[41] Andre F, Ismaila N, Allison KH, Barlow WE, Collyar DE, Damodaran S, et al. Biomarkers for adjuvant endocrine and chemotherapy in early-stage breast cancer: ASCO guideline update. Journal of Clinical Oncology. 2022;**40**(16):1816-1837. DOI: 10.1200/JCO.22.00069

[42] Cho JY, Lim JY, Cheong JH, Park YY, Yoon SL, Kim SM, et al. Gene expression signature-based prognostic risk score in gastric cancer. Clinical Cancer Research. 2011;**17**(7):1850-1857. DOI: 10.1158/1078-0432.CCR-10-2180

[43] Wu Y, Grabsch H, Ivanova T, Tan IB, Murray J, Ooi CH, et al. Comprehensive genomic meta-analysis identifies intra-tumoural stroma as a predictor of survival in patients with gastric cancer. Gut. 2013;**62**(8):1100-1111. DOI: 10.1136/gutjnl-2011-301373

[44] Park S, Karalis JD, Hong C, Clemenceau JR, Porembka MR, Kim IH, et al. ACTA2 expression predicts survival and is associated with response to immune checkpoint inhibitors in gastric cancer. Clinical Cancer Research. 2023;**29**(6):1077-1085. DOI: 10.1158/1078-0432.CCR-22-1897

[45] Sohn BH, Hwang JE, Jang HJ, Lee HS, Oh SC, Shim JJ, et al. Clinical significance of four molecular subtypes of gastric Cancer identified by the cancer genome atlas project. Clinical Cancer Research. 2017;**23**(15):4441-4449. DOI: 10.1158/1078-0432.CCR-16-2211

[46] Jiang Y, Zhang Q, Hu Y, Li T, Yu J, Zhao L, et al. ImmunoScore signature: A prognostic and predictive tool in gastric cancer. Annals of Surgery. 2018;**267**(3):504-513. DOI: 10.1097/SLA.0000000000002116

[47] Cheong JH, Yang HK, Kim H, Kim WH, Kim YW, Kook MC, et al. Predictive test for chemotherapy response in resectable gastric cancer: A multi-cohort, retrospective analysis. The Lancet Oncology. 2018;**19**(5):629-638. DOI: 10.1016/S1470-2045(18)30108-6

[48] Kerr DJ, Yang L. Personalising cancer medicine with prognostic markers. eBioMedicine. 2021;**72**:103577. DOI: 10.1016/j.ebiom.2021.103577

[49] Choi YY, Jang E, Seo WJ, Son T, Kim HI, Kim H, et al. Modification of the TNM staging system for stage II/III gastric cancer based on a prognostic single patient classifier algorithm. Journal of Gastric Cancer. 2018;**18**(2):142-151. DOI: 10.5230/jgc.2018.18.e14

[50] Choi YY, Jang E, Kim H, Kim KM, Noh SH, Sohn TS, et al. Single patient classifier as a prognostic biomarker in pT1N1 gastric cancer: Results from two large Korean cohorts. Chinese Journal of Cancer Research. 2021;**33**(5):583-591. DOI: 10.21147/j.issn.1000-9604.2021.05.05

[51] Kim YM, Kwon IG, Choi SH, Noh SH, Chun J, Youn YH, et al. SFRP4 and CDX1 are predictive genes for Extragastric recurrence of early gastric cancer after curative resection. Journal of Clinical Medicine. 2022;**11**(11):3072. DOI: 10.3390/jcm11113072

[52] National Comprehensive Cancer Network. Clinical Practice Guidelines in Oncology. Gastric Cancer. Version 1. 2023. Available from: https://www.nccn.org/professionals/physician_gls/pdf/gastric.pdf (Accessed: July 12, 2023]

[53] Amin MB, Edge S, Greene F, Byrd DR, Brookland RK, Washington MK, et al., editors. AJCC Cancer Staging Manual. 8th ed. Springer International Publishing

and American Joint Commission on Cancer; 2017

[54] Simon RM, Paik S, Hayes DF. Use of archived specimens in evaluation of prognostic and predictive biomarkers. Journal of the National Cancer Institute. 2009;**101**(21):1446-1452. DOI: 10.1093/jnci/djp335

[55] Imfinzi (durvalumab) Plus Chemotherapy Significantly Improved Pathologic Complete Response in Gastric and Gastroesophageal Junction Cancers in MATTERHORN Phase III trial. News Release. AstraZeneca. 2023. Available from: https://www.astrazeneca-us.com/media/press-releases/2023/imfinzi-durvalumab-plus-chemotherapy-significantly-improved-pathologic-complete-response-in-gastric-and-gastroesophageal-junction-cancers-in-matterhorn-phase-iii-trial-06022023.html [Accessed: June 07, 2023]

[56] Zhao JJ, Yap DWT, Chan YH, Tan BKJ, Teo CB, Syn NL, et al. Low programmed death-ligand 1-expressing subgroup outcomes of first-line immune checkpoint inhibitors in gastric or Esophageal adenocarcinoma. Journal of Clinical Oncology. 2022;**40**(4):392-402. DOI: 10.1200/JCO.21.01862

[57] Chao J, Fuchs CS, Shitara K, Tabernero J, Muro K, Van Cutsem E, et al. Assessment of Pembrolizumab therapy for the treatment of microsatellite instability-high gastric or gastroesophageal junction cancer among patients in the KEYNOTE-059, KEYNOTE-061, and KEYNOTE-062 clinical trials. JAMA Oncology. 2021;**7**(6):895-902. DOI: 10.1001/jamaoncol.2021.0275

[58] Shitara K, Özgüroğlu M, Bang YJ, Di Bartolomeo M, Mandalà M, Ryu MH, et al. Molecular determinants of clinical outcomes with pembrolizumab versus paclitaxel in a randomized, open-label, phase III trial in patients with gastroesophageal adenocarcinoma. Annals of Oncology. 2021;**32**(9):1127-1136. DOI: 10.1016/j.annonc.2021.05.803

[59] Lee KW, Van Cutsem E, Bang YJ, Fuchs CS, Kudaba I, Garrido M, et al. Association of Tumor Mutational Burden with efficacy of Pembrolizumab±chemotherapy as first-line therapy for gastric cancer in the phase III KEYNOTE-062 study. Clinical Cancer Research. 2022;**28**(16):3489-3498. DOI: 10.1158/1078-0432.CCR-22-0121

[60] Kim ST, Cristescu R, Bass AJ, Kim KM, Odegaard JI, Kim K, et al. Comprehensive molecular characterization of clinical responses to PD-1 inhibition in metastatic gastric cancer. Nature Medicine. 2018;**24**(9):1449-1458. DOI: 10.1038/s41591-018-0101-z

[61] Smyth EC, Wotherspoon A, Peckitt C, Gonzalez D, Hulkki-Wilson S, Eltahir Z, et al. Mismatch repair deficiency, microsatellite instability, and survival: An exploratory analysis of the Medical Research Council adjuvant gastric infusional chemotherapy (MAGIC) trial. JAMA Oncology. 2017;**3**(9):1197-1203. DOI: 10.1001/jamaoncol.2016.6762

[62] Choi YY, Kim H, Shin SJ, Kim HY, Lee J, Yang HK, et al. Microsatellite instability and programmed cell death-ligand 1 expression in stage II/III gastric cancer: Post hoc analysis of the CLASSIC randomized controlled study. Annals of Surgery. 2019;**270**(2):309-316. DOI: 10.1097/SLA.0000000000002803

[63] Shitara K, Di Bartolomeo M, Mandala M, Ryu MH, Caglevic C, Olesinski T, et al. Association between gene expression signatures and clinical outcomes of pembrolizumab

versus paclitaxel in advanced gastric cancer: Exploratory analysis from the randomized, controlled, phase III KEYNOTE-061 trial. Journal for Immunotherapy of Cancer. 2023;**11**(6):e006920. DOI: 10.1136/jitc-2023-006920

[64] Shitara K, Lordick F, Bang YJ, Enzinger P, Ilson D, Shah MA, et al. Zolbetuximab plus mFOLFOX6 in patients with CLDN18.2-positive, HER2-negative, untreated, locally advanced unresectable or metastatic gastric or gastro-oesophageal junction adenocarcinoma (SPOTLIGHT): A multicentre, randomised, double-blind, phase 3 trial. Lancet. 2023;**401**(10389):1655-1668. DOI: 10.1016/S0140-6736(23)00620-7

[65] Shah MA, Shitara K, Ajani JA, Bang YJ, Enzinger P, Ilson D, et al. Zolbetuximab plus CAPOX in CLDN18.2-positive gastric or gastroesophageal junction adenocarcinoma: The randomized, phase 3 GLOW trial. Nature Medicine. 2023;**29**(8):2133-2141. DOI: 10.1038/s41591-023-02465-7

[66] Coati I, Lotz G, Fanelli GN, Brignola S, Lanza C, Cappellesso R, et al. Claudin-18 expression in oesophagogastric adenocarcinomas: A tissue microarray study of 523 molecularly profiled cases. British Journal of Cancer. 2019;**121**(3):257-263. DOI: 10.1038/s41416-019-0508-4

[67] Rohde C, Yamaguchi R, Mukhina S, Sahin U, Itoh K, Türeci Ö. Comparison of Claudin 18.2 expression in primary tumors and lymph node metastases in Japanese patients with gastric adenocarcinoma. Japanese Journal of Clinical Oncology. 2019;**49**(9):870-876. DOI: 10.1093/jjco/hyz068

[68] Xu B, Liu F, Liu Q, Shi T, Wang Z, Wu N, et al. Highly expressed Claudin18.2 as a potential therapeutic target in advanced gastric signet-ring cell carcinoma (SRCC). Journal of Gastrointestinal Oncology. 2020;**11**(6):1431-1439. DOI: 10.21037/jgo-20-344

[69] Kubota Y, Kawazoe A, Mishima S, Nakamura Y, Kotani D, Kuboki Y, et al. Comprehensive clinical and molecular characterization of claudin 18.2 expression in advanced gastric or gastroesophageal junction cancer. ESMO Open. 2023;**8**(1):100762. DOI: 10.1016/j.esmoop.2022.100762

[70] Wainberg ZA, Enzinger PC, Kang YK, Qin S, Yamaguchi K, Kim IH, et al. Bemarituzumab in patients with FGFR2b-selected gastric or gastro-oesophageal junction adenocarcinoma (FIGHT): A randomised, double-blind, placebo-controlled, phase 2 study. The Lancet Oncology. 2022;**23**(11):1430-1440. DOI: 10.1016/S1470-2045(22)00603-9

[71] Kim HS, Kim JH, Jang HJ. Pathologic and prognostic impacts of FGFR2 amplification in gastric cancer: A meta-analysis and systemic review. Journal of Cancer. 2019;**10**(11):2560-2567. DOI: 10.7150/jca.29184

[72] Jeong MH, Park SY, Lee SH, Seo J, Yoo JY, Park SH, et al. EPB41L5 mediates TGFβ-induced metastasis of gastric cancer. Clinical Cancer Research. 2019;**25**(12):3617-3629. DOI: 10.1158/1078-0432.CCR-18-2959

[73] Kim BK, Kim DM, Park H, Kim SK, Hwang MA, Lee J, et al. Synaptotagmin 11 scaffolds MKK7-JNK signaling process to promote stem-like molecular subtype gastric cancer oncogenesis. Journal of Experimental & Clinical Cancer Research. 2022;**41**(1):212. DOI: 10.1186/s13046-022-02420-3

[74] Lee J, Kim H, Lee JE, Shin SJ, Oh S, Kwon G, et al. Selective cytotoxicity of

the NAMPT inhibitor FK866 toward gastric cancer cells with markers of the epithelial-mesenchymal transition, due to loss of NAPRT. Gastroenterology. 2018;**155**(3):799-814.e13. DOI: 10.1053/j.gastro.2018.05.024

[75] Park KC, Kim JM, Kim SY, Kim SM, Lim JH, Kim MK, et al. PMCA inhibition reverses drug resistance in clinically refractory cancer patient-derived models. BMC Medicine. 2023;**21**(1):38. DOI: 10.1186/s12916-023-02727-8

[76] Yoon BK, Kim H, Oh TG, Oh SK, Jo S, Kim M, et al. PHGDH preserves one-carbon cycle to confer metabolic plasticity in chemoresistant gastric cancer during nutrient stress. Proceedings of the National Academy of Sciences of the United States of America. 2023;**120**(21):e2217826120. DOI: 10.1073/pnas.2217826120

[77] Lee JY, Nam M, Son HY, Hyun K, Jang SY, Kim JW, et al. Polyunsaturated fatty acid biosynthesis pathway determines ferroptosis sensitivity in gastric cancer. Proceedings of the National Academy of Sciences of the United States of America. 2020;**117**(51):32433-32442. DOI: 10.1073/pnas.2006828117

Chapter 5

New Approaches in Gastric Cancer Immunotherapy

Pegah Mousavi, Ali Ahmadi, Shakila Behzadifar, Javad Mohammadnejad and Seyed Mohammad Hosseini

Abstract

Cancer has an inferior prognosis in most cases and is often challenging to treat. Gastric cancer (GC), which is among leading causes of the top five malignant tumor deaths worldwide and whose incidence is increasing every day, is no exception. GC is frequently diagnosed at a progressive or metastatic stage of the disease. At this stage, the clinical effectiveness of conventional treatments such as surgery and chemotherapy is limited, and the median overall survival is reduced to only about a few months. The tumor microenvironment (TME) and the specific conditions that govern it, concurrently with multiple mutations, have significantly increased the resistance of cancer cells. However, the study of molecular biology, cell signaling pathways, and immune system function provides a new approach using immunotherapy such as immune inhibitors, T cell transfer therapy, monoclonal antibodies (mAbs), therapeutic vaccines, etc. to overcome cancer resistance. In addition, the use of nanoparticles (NPs), especially theranostic NPs permits for better monitoring of the response during treatment, and its combination with immunotherapy, promising strategies for providing a new treatment. This chapter provides an overview of these new advances in treating GC cancer.

Keywords: gastric cancer, immunotherapy, Theranostic, precision medicine, tumor microenvironment

1. Introduction

Gastric cancer (GC) is the fifth most prevalent cancer and the third leading cause of cancer-related death. The highest incidence of GC occurs in East Asia, followed by Eastern and Central Europe, and it is more prevalent in men. Because of the poor prognosis, many GC cases are diagnosed at advanced stages, limiting treatment options, and increasing mortality [1, 2]. Exposure to Hp, dietary risk factors, obesity, tobacco, meat, alcohol consumption, genetics, and socioeconomic status play a role in its development. More than 95% of GCs are adenocarcinomas classified by anatomic location and histologic type (**Table 1**) [3–9]. GC is generally treated with a combination of surgery, endoscopy, and chemotherapy, which can have side effects that can have a substantial influence on patients' quality of life. The physical removal of

Gastric cancer			
Anatomic location		Histological type (Lauren classification)	
Cardia (Proximal)	Non-cardia (Distal)	Diffuse	Intestinal
• Mainly in developed countries (more common in Western countries) • Risk factors: smoking (also in combination with drinking), consumption of food containing carcinogens, and exposure to Epstein-Barr virus (EBV) • less lymph-node metastasis, good differentiation, Bigger in size, poor differentiation • Molecular pathology: CIN and EBV type • Survival: Higher 5-year survival rate	• Mainly in developing countries (more common in East Asian populations) • Risk factors: *H. pylori* infection (strong correlation), smoking, high-salt diet, food with carcinogens • more lymph-node metastasis, Bigger in size, poor differentiation • Molecular pathology: MSI type • Survival: Lower 5-year survival rate	• Is correlated with non-cardia • prevalent in low-risk areas • mainly associated with heritable genetic abnormalities • frequently occurs in the gastric antrum • diffusely infiltrating the gastric wall in a desmoplastic stroma • characterized by poorly differentiated and discohesive tumor cells that may have either a signet-ring or non-signet-ring morphology. • tumor cells lack adhesion	• Is correlated with cardio • more frequently in high-risk areas • mainly found in the cardia and gastric fundus • most commonly occurs in elderly male • is more associated with environmental factors • tumor cells exhibit adhesion • are arranged in tubular or glandular formations • affects the gastric antrum

Table 1.
The categorization and features of adenocarcinoma in GC.

malignant tissue is a key component of stomach cancer therapy. Minimally invasive procedures like laparoscopic surgery and endoscopy are used for early detection and removal of tumors. Endoscopic mucosal resection (EMR) and endoscopic submucosal dissection (ESD) are two endoscopic methods routinely used to remove early-stage stomach tumors. Despite its serious side effects, chemotherapy is still used as a treatment for advanced stomach cancer. Combination chemotherapy treatments have been found to enhance survival rates. Nausea, vomiting, exhaustion, and hair loss are some of the side effects of chemotherapy, which can be severe. On the other hand, the tumor microenvironment (TME) and multi-drug resistance by mutations in cancer cells and ABC family pumps (ATP-binding cassette) reduce its therapeutic effect. New treatment methods like immunotherapy and nanoparticles are being used to target and eliminate cancer cells. In the following sections, we will discuss all the above in detail [10–14].

2. Tumor microenvironment

The extracellular matrix that encompasses a range of cells, including cancer cells, cancer-associated fibroblasts (CAFs), pericytes, and other immune cells, is known as the TEM. The milieu around tumors, primarily made up of stromal and immunological cells, continuously affects the tumor cells [15].

2.1 Cancer-associated fibroblasts (CAFs)

About 70% of the cells in tumor tissues are CAFs, which are significant elements of malignancies such as GC [16]. They control processes such as angiogenesis, chemoresistance, and metabolic reprogramming, making them crucial in determining the spread of cancer. CAFs particularly control GC cell signaling, encouraging migration, invasion, and proliferation. They can also control immune cell activity and induce hypoxic or angiogenic circumstances through various signaling pathways. Furthermore, by secreting cytokines and chemokines, expressing cell surface receptor proteins, and remodeling the extracellular matrix (ECM), CAFs can control immune cell activity and their location and movement within the TME [17–21]. Subtypes of CAFs that co-expressed FAP and INHBA markers were discovered to be connected with a more advanced stage in the TME of GC. Myofibroblasts, pericytes, eCAFs, and iCAFs are the four main subpopulations of fibroblasts that were found to contribute to diffuse GC carcinogenesis. iCAFs contribute to diffuse GC carcinogenesis and may be implicated in DGC's de novo carcinogenesis. CAFs not only shape the ECM but also supply signaling molecules that change the behavior of tumors and promote tumor survival. The Wnt/PCP signaling pathway is critical for invasion and metastasis in GC. CAFs generate WNT5A, which is the essential PCP ligand, and GC cells respond to this signal by enhancing polarized migration. CAFs secrete certain biological molecules such as Transforming Growth Factor-β (TGF-β), IL-6, and Epidermal growth factor (EGF) to promote tumor malignant phenotype, which includes tumor neovascularization and immune evasion, ultimately resulting in tumor deterioration. CAFs can also control tumor metabolism by creating an acidic milieu that inhibits the function of immune cells. Furthermore, tumor cells can exploit the metabolites of pyruvate and lactic acid generated by CAFs as nutrients to promote their proliferation [22–27].

2.2 Immune cells

For immune editing and immunosurveillance against cancer, the host immunological response is essential. Target cells for immunotherapy include natural killer (NK) cells, dendritic cells (DCs), tumor-associated macrophages (TAMs), tumor-associated neutrophils (TANs), myeloid-derived suppressor cells (MDSCs), T cells, B cells, and regulatory T cells (Tregs). These cells are found in the TEM [28–30]. Through a variety of tumor cells can avoid immune system recognition and elimination. M2 TAMs, N2 TANs, MDSCs, regulatory B cells (Bregs), effector Tregs (eTregs), and inhibitory targets on different immune cells are among them that are important in tumor immune escape while tumor-infiltrating DCs, NK, M1 TAMs, and N1 TANs are helpful in anti-tumor immunity (**Figure 1**) [30].

2.2.1 Dendritic cells (DCs)

Dendritic cells play a crucial role in activating T cells and bridging innate and adaptive immunity. Maintaining a sufficient density of mature DCs within tumors is essential for prolonged life of patients with advanced GC. There are two types of DCs: conventional DCs (cDCs; sometimes called myeloid DCs) and plasmacytoid DCs (pDCs) pDCs have gained interest in recent years for their ability to present antigens, secrete cytokines, and promote the proliferation and functionality of immune cells [31, 32].

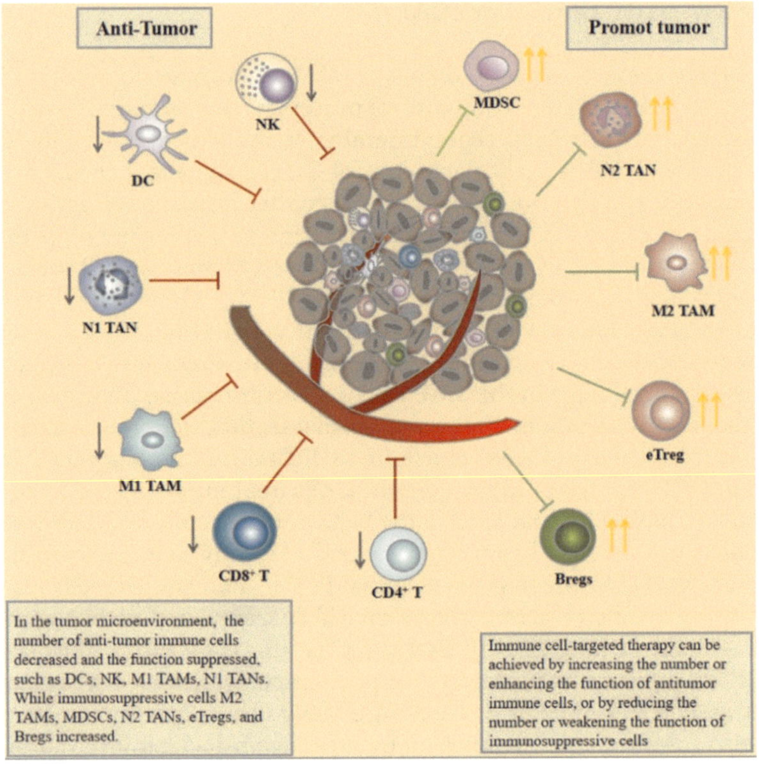

Figure 1.
Immune cell-targeted treatment can be accomplished by either boosting anti-tumor immune cell counts or functions or by decreasing immunosuppressive cell counts or functions [30]. Copyright 2022 Frontiersin.

2.2.2 Natural killer cells

NK cells play a crucial role in regulating the immune system against cancer cells and intracellular viruses. They identify tumor cells via NKG2D and eliminate them using perforin, death receptor signaling, or granzymes that generate cytokines and chemokines [33–35]. NK cells contain inhibitory receptors on their surface, which allows tumor cells to connect to them and evade NK cell killing. On the other hand, excess TGF-β, together with other chemokines and anti-inflammatory cytokines, can prevent NK cell activation in the TEM; produce some immunosuppressive factors, and downregulate NK cell activating receptors such as NKp30, NKp44, NKG2D, and CD16 as well as co-receptors including NKp80 and DNAM-1. It also upregulates checkpoint receptors such as TIGIT, TIM-3, LAG-3, and PD-1 [36–38].

2.2.3 Tumor-associated macrophages

Macrophages are a type of immune cell that infiltrate solid tumors. They are divided into two subgroups: M1 and M2. M1 macrophages have proinflammatory effects and produce High amounts of TNF-α, IFN-γ, IL-1β, IL-6, IL-12, CXCL9, and CXCL10 that stimulate type 1 (polarizing and recruiting Th1) responses aiding in the elimination of infections and tumor cells. On the other hand, M2 macrophages have anti-inflammatory effects and produce TGF-β1 (TGF-β1), IL-4, and IL-10 that have tumorigenic qualities [39–42]. Macrophages play a crucial role in gastric inflammation during *H. pylori* infection. In GC tissue, macrophages are more abundant and their gene expression patterns are diverse. Macrophage-GC cell crosstalk contributes to the development of an immunosuppressive milieu and the progression of GC. M2 features are linked to a poor prognosis in many tumor types [43–47].

2.2.4 Tumor-associated neutrophils

As the initial line of defense against infection and inflammation, neutrophils play a crucial role in Innate immune responses. Neutrophils are associated with a worse prognosis in GC patients and are abundant in GC tissue [48–50]. Neutrophils are one kind of immune cell that promotes angiogenesis and inhibits the anti-tumor immune response, which contributes to the development of tumors [32]. GC-derived GM-CSF suppresses T-cell activity to advance GC by activating neutrophils and eliciting PD-L1 expression via the JK-STAT3 signaling pathway. Additionally, TANs secrete cytokines that aid in GC invasion and migration, including IL-1β, IL-6, IL-8, IL-17a, and IL-23 [48, 51, 52].

2.2.5 Myeloid-derived suppressor cells

The primary role of myeloid-derived cells, or MDSCs, is immunosuppression. They are a very diverse collection of cells. Malignant tumors with MDSC growth had a poor prognosis and were linked to treatment resistance. Increased MDSC levels were linked to later tumor stages, a worse prognosis, increased mortality, and a higher chance of tumor progression and recurrence in GC patient's survival [53–55]. These relationships were also seen between MDSC levels and the cancer stage. MDSCs are involved in the production of immunosuppressive TME as well as the advancement and metastasis of tumors (**Figure 2**) [57–59].

2.2.6 B cells

In addition to acting as APCs, B cells also create and ingest cytokines including IL-6, IFN-γ, and TNF-a, which help to develop CD4$^+$ and memory T cells [60]. Research has demonstrated that effector T cells, NK cells, and TAMs, as well as T cells and other immune cells, are the primary mediators of antitumoral activity, which is inhibited by a subset of B regulatory cells called Bregs [61].

2.2.7 T cells

T lymphocytes come in different varieties: helper T cells (CD4$^+$ cells), Tregs, and cytotoxic T cells (CD8$^+$ cells). The TME's CD8$^+$ T cell subset is widely regarded as having immunological activation to produce antitumor effects, and the prognosis and treatment results of GC malignancies are strongly correlated with the subsets' variety and density. Tumor prognoses vary depending on different T cell subsets. T-cell subsets that are advantageous to the prognosis and survival of GC include those with a high T helper (TH)1/TH2 ratio, high CD45RO memory T cells, and high levels of infiltration of CD8$^+$ and CD4$^+$ T cells [62–64].

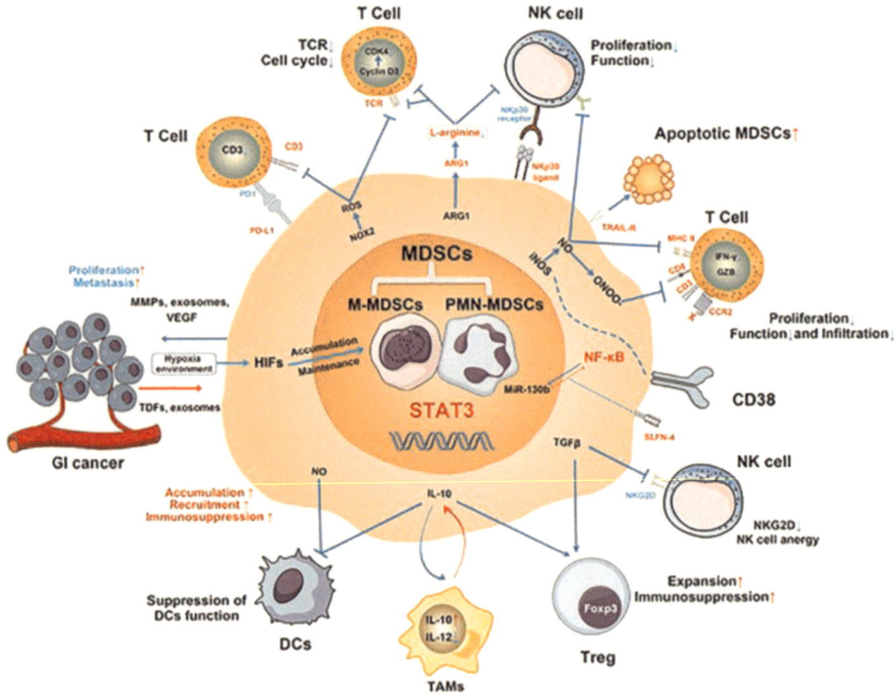

Figure 2.
The processes via which gastrointestinal (GI) cancer is immunosuppressed by MDSC. MDSCs block the activity of DCs, prevent DCs from presenting antigens to CD4$^+$ *T cells, repress the growth and function of NK and T cells, decrease CD8*$^+$ *T-cell infiltration, support M2 macrophage development, and stimulate the expansion and immunosuppression of Tregs. Moreover, nitric oxide (NO) generation and TGF-β-induced suppression of NKG2D have an impact on ADCC function and NK cell anergy, respectively. To encourage the proliferation and metastasis of GI cancer cells, MDSCs produce exosomes, matrix metalloproteinases (MMPs), and VEGF [56]. Copyright 2021 Wiley.*

2.2.8 Regulatory T cells

From 5–10% of peripheral CD4$^+$ T cells are Tregs, which are responsible for maintaining immunological tolerance linked to tumor immunity. Numerous investigations have documented the significance of Tregs as a constituent of immune-suppressive cells, which expedite the growth of tumors in diverse malignancies by inhibiting T cell proliferation, antigen presentation, and cytokine generation. Based on how FOXP3 and CD45RA are expressed, TME Tregs may be divided into three groups: effector Tregs (eTregs) (FOXP3highCD45RA$^-$), naïve Tregs (FOXP3lowCD45RA$^+$), and non-Tregs (FOXP3lowCD45RA$^-$). Non-Tregs can release pro-inflammatory cytokines but are unable to have an inhibitory impact. The function of eTregs is persistent and has substantial suppressive activity, while naïve Tregs only exhibit mild suppression [65–67]. In **Figure 3**, the various T cells, B cells, and Tregs are discussed concerning the GC microenvironment; **Figure 4** also illustrates the significance of TAMs, NK cells, DC cells, and neutrophils in this context.

We have summarized the findings of various studies to enhance understanding regarding the role of immune cells, such as T cells, TAM cells, B cells, NK cells, DC cells, neutrophils, and cytokines secreted by stromal cells in GC progression. You can find this summary in **Table 2** for your better understanding.

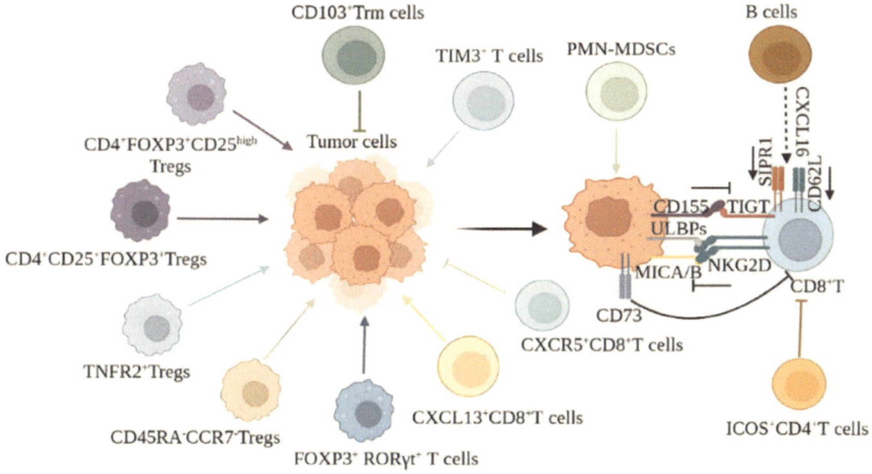

Figure 3.
The functions of various B cells, Tregs, and T cells in the stomach cancer microenvironment. In GC, certain Tregs and dysfunctional CTLs accelerate disease progression, while specific T cell subsets indicate poor outcomes. Conversely, CXCR5+ CD8+ T cells and CD103+ Trm cells are associated with better survival. PMN-MDSCs contribute to immunosuppression as cancer develops. Elevated CD73 expression in tumors enhances CD8+ T cell infiltration. Reduced expression of homing receptors in Aim2−/− mice leads to increased gastric CD8+ T cell frequency and metaplasia. Higher levels of NKG2D correlate with improved survival, as it interacts with tumor cells' MICA/B and ULBPs. CD155 on tumor cells inhibits TIGIT+ CD8 T cells' glucose uptake, diminishing their function. ICOS+ CD4 + T cells hinder CD8+ T cell proliferation, hastening disease advancement [29]. Copyright 2023 Springer.

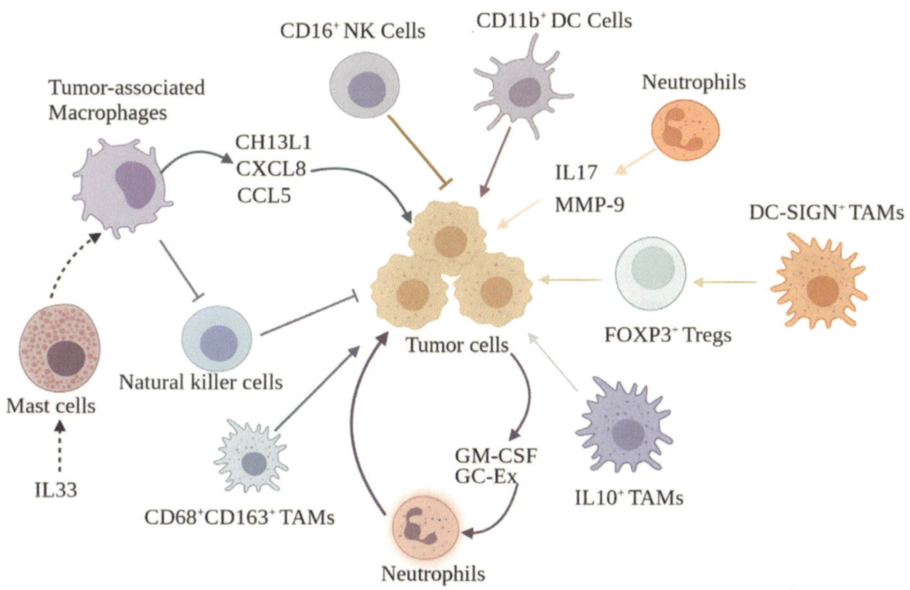

Figure 4.
The functions of DC cells, neutrophils, NK cells, and TAMs in the GC microenvironment. In gastric cancer microenvironment, TAMs release immunosuppressive chemicals like CH13HL1, CXCL8, and CCL5, promoting tumor growth. Neutrophils' secretion of MMP-9 and IL-17 correlates with poor prognosis. IL-33-driven mast cell buildup, facilitated by macrophage mobilization, contributes to GC progression in certain animal models. High levels of CD68+, CD163+, and IL10+ macrophages correlate with decreased survival rates. DC-SIGN+ macrophages elevate FOXP3 Treg levels, associated with lower overall survival. TAMs reduce NK cell percentage and function, while NK cells express CD16 and exhibit direct antitumor effects. Poor prognosis in GC patients is linked to high CD11b levels in DC cells, which lowers MHC class II expression. Neutrophils, driven by GC cell-derived exosomes and GM-CSF, promote tumor migration and enhance their own survival [29]. Copyright 2023 Springer.

Immune cells	Cancer type	Functions	Ref.
Dendritic cells			
DC cells	GC	foreseen prognosis is unsatisfactory	[68]
Plasmacytoid DC cells	GC	Improved the efficiency of cancer treatments	[31]
Natural killer cells			
NK cells	GC	Foresaw a more satisfactory 5-year survival rate compared to lysis activity of less than 25%	[69]
NK cells	GC	Effectively, trastuzumab-targeted tumor cells with a potent killing	[70]
NK cells	GC	Compared to low NK cell density has a more favorable prognosis GC	[71]
NK cells	GC	Survival is predicted to be longer	[72]
NK cells	GC	Tumor cells exhibit limited immune evasion.	[73]
NK cells	GC	Predicted better OS	[74]
High-affinity NK cells	GC	Induced direct antitumor effects	[75]
Tumor-associated macrophages			
TAMs	GC	Prompted HMGB1 expression contributes to chemoresistance to 5-Fu	[76]
TAMs	GC	Boosted PD-L1 expression and tumor metastasis	[77]
TAMs	GC	Impaired NK cell proportion and function	[78]
TAMs	GC	Enhanced DNMT1 and low GSN expression to promote tumor growth	[79]
DC-SIGN+ TAMs	GC	Indicated poor OS and resistance to ACT such as 5-Fu	[80]
CD68+ CD163+ not MARCO+ TAMs	Gastroesophageal adenocarcinoma	Indicted poor survival	[81]
IL10+ TAMs	GC	Promoted regulatory T cell infiltration and CD8+ T cell dysfunction	[82]
Neutrophils			
Neutrophils	GC	Induced tumor migration	[83]
Neutrophils	GC	Executed Immunosuppression	[49]
Neutrophils in the peripheral blood	GC	Indicated poor prognosis	[84]
Myeloid-derived Suppressor cells			
PMN-MDSCs	GC	Executed immunosuppressive function	[85]
T cells			

Immune cells	Cancer type	Functions	Ref.
CD8+ T cells	Gastric and gastroesophageal junction (G/GEJ) adenocarcinomas	Shortened PFS and OS	[86]
CD8+ T cells	GC with high CD73 expression	The phenotype of the $CD8^+$ T cells indicated that they were dysfunctional.	[87]
CXCR5 + CD8+ T cells	GC with TNM II + III stage	Benefited from ACT	[88]
CXCL13+ CD8+ T cells	GC	Indicated poor prognosis	[89]
(ICOS+) CD4+ T cells	GC	Impeded the proliferation of CD8+ T cells	[90]
Foxp3+ RORγt+ T cells	GC	Predicted poor overall survival	[91]
Tumor-infiltrating γδT cells	GC with TNM II + III stage	Benefited from 5-Fu ACT	[92]
CD69+ CD103+ Trm	Gastric adenocarcinoma	Predicted better survival	[93]
HLA-1-preserved type/PDL1+	Microsatellite-unstable GC tumors	Indicated good prognosis	[94]
TIM3+ cells	GC	Had poorer OS and disease-free survival (DFS)	[95]
Regulatory T Cells			
TNFR2+ Tregs	GC	Promoted the GC progression	[96]
CD4 + CD25 + FOXP3 + Tregs	GC	Helped immune-suppressive roles of Tregs	[97]
CD45RA − CCR7− Tregs	GC	Exerted immunosuppression	[98]
CD4+ FOXP3+ CD25high Tregs	GC	Exerted Immunosuppression	[99]
FOXP3+ Tregs	Stage I–II GC patients	Foreseen more acceptable prognosis	[100]
B cells			
B regulatory cells	GC	Inhibited antitumoral activity	[61]
CD20+ B cells	GC	Prospered disease-free survival and overall survival rate	[101]
Cytokines or chemokines	Cancer type	Functions	Ref
CCL28	GC	Drove GC tumor progression	[102]
IL-9	GC	Achieved additional benefits from 5-Fu-based adjuvant chemotherapy and Lengthy OS	[103]
IL-15	GC	Promoted tumor progression	[104]
IL-17	GC	Benefited from adjuvant chemo-therapy	[105]
IL17B	GC	Accelerated cancer stem cell tumorigenesis and self-renewal	[106]

Table 2.
A review of the immune system's role in GC disease progression, by different immune cells, cytokines, and chemokines.

3. Resistance to the treatment of gastric cancer

GC is known for its resistance to standard treatments like chemotherapy and radiotherapy. Immunotherapy is a promising approach, but its effectiveness is often hindered by TEM of GC. Surgical resection with lymphadenectomy is the primary treatment strategy for GC. Surgery is the primary option for GC due to its resistance to chemotherapy and radiation [107, 108]. The TEM in GC is distinct from normal tissue, leading to fluctuations in glucose, lactate, oxygen tension, and acidic pH. Glycolysis leads to lactic acid production and subsequent tumor acidosis. Aggressive tumors rely heavily on glycolysis for energy production, even in the presence of adequate oxygen, exacerbating the acidic environment [109, 110].

3.1 Hypoxia

GC microenvironment is characterized notably by hypoxia and inflammation. Hypoxia, defined as a reduction in normal tissue oxygen levels, emerges due to rapid tumor cell proliferation surpassing the oxygen delivery capabilities of existing blood vessels. This condition triggers a series of cellular responses in tumor cells, enabling them to adapt and thrive in this low-oxygen environment. These cells undergo a range of molecular and physiological adaptations under hypoxic conditions, which often include upregulation of hypoxia-inducible factors (HIFs), alterations in metabolic pathways such as a shift towards anaerobic glycolysis, and the activation of survival and proliferative signaling pathways [111–113]. hypoxia in TEM is linked to poor clinical outcomes and treatment resistance in GC. Hypoxia triggers hypoxia-inducible factor-1 (HIF-1), which regulates the expression of many cancer-promoting molecules. HIF-1 is crucial in promoting angiogenesis, which is vital for tumor growth and spread in hypoxic conditions. Hypoxia also triggers the production of immune checkpoint molecules like PD-L1, which naturally slow down T-cell activity. Overexpression of PD-L1 hinders the effectiveness of immunotherapies, like checkpoint inhibitors, that aim to activate the immune system against cancer cells. Hypoxic GC cells show higher levels of PD-L1 expression, which contributes to the evasion of immune surveillance [30, 114–116].

3.2 Oxidative stress

Oxidative stress affects the resistance of GC to immunotherapy. In an oxidative stress state is a lack of balance between the body's antioxidant defenses and the production of reactive oxygen species (ROS). High levels of ROS in GC can lead to genetic mutations, cancer cell proliferation, and metastasis, which often result in an increased resistance to cancer therapy, including immunotherapy [117–119]. For instance, oxidative stress can impair the effectiveness of T cells, a crucial part of the immune response in immunotherapy. However, targeting oxidative stress in treating GC is challenging due to the complex role of ROS in cancer biology, where it can both promote and inhibit tumor growth. It also requires sophisticated techniques and a deep understanding of tumor physiology to accurately assess and modulate oxidative stress levels within tumors [120, 121].

3.3 Acidosis

Changes in metabolic processes, specifically the Warburg effect, cause acidosis in tumors. The cancer cells consume glucose through glycolysis instead of oxidative phosphorylation, which results in the production of lactic acid. This, in turn, lowers the pH of the environment surrounding the tumor [122, 123]. This can impair the effectiveness of immunotherapies by inhibiting the function and survival of T cells and upregulating immune checkpoint molecules. The acidic environment also inhibits the effector functions of activated CD8+ T-cells. The study of Wu shows that acidic paracortical zones in lymph nodes inhibit the effector functions of activated CD8+ T-cells and hinder T-cell glycolysis. This low pH, is a result of the acid inhibition of monocarboxylate transporters (MCTs), leading to a decrease in the glycolytic rate [124]. Despite this, the acidic environment does not prevent the initial activation of native T-cells by DCs. Low pH conditions reduce cytokine production and proliferative capacity of T cells, which are crucial for their cancer-fighting abilities [125, 126]. Acidosis can also upregulate PD-L1 expression, contributing to the resistance to immunotherapy [127, 128].

4. New approaches in cancer immunotherapy

Despite advancements in GC treatment, there's debate on the most effective approach. Multimodal treatments have improved patient survival, but over 70% of patients cannot be rescued. The side effects of therapy can lower the quality of life, which can impact the outcome. This fact has made researchers explore alternative approaches to managing GC [129, 130]. For GC treatment, there are several therapeutic methods with a different level of invasiveness from surgery to adjuvant therapies yet surgery is considered the priority therapy. Although, whether preoperative or postoperative, has shown improvement in the overall outcome of GC treatment, each of the conventional therapies comes with a spectrum of complications, ranging from severe to mild. Despite the radiotherapy, chemotherapy, and chemoradiotherapy have advanced, surgical resection remains the primary treatment option for GC. However, it is a high-risk procedure with significant morbidity and mortality, especially in elderly patients, has a lower tolerance for anesthesia and surgery due to a decline in organ function and an increase in internal diseases. While postoperative mortality has decreased by more than 50% in four decades, significant surgical morbidity following gastrectomy continues to pose challenges [131, 132]. Chemotherapy has been found to have comparable or better survival rates compared to surgeries for GC. Palliative chemotherapy enhances survival rates without impacting the quality of life significantly. Nausea, vomiting, and diarrhea are some common side effects However, acute chemotherapy complications like GI hemorrhage, perforation, nausea, vomiting, diarrhea, and typhlitis, from neutropenia by chemotherapy manifest as localized inflammation in the caecal wall [133–135]. Other approaches, such as radiation therapy, have been investigated to improve outcomes. However, radiation therapy can have severe side effects such as skin problems, diarrhea, fatigue, and low blood cell counts. Patients may encounter GI side effects [136, 137].

4.1 Novel immunotherapy methods

Immunotherapy emerged as a potent clinical approach to cancer therapy. The quantity of approved immunotherapy drugs has been steadily rising and there are also numerous treatments undergoing preclinical development and clinical trials. Immunotherapies for GI cancers include a range of approaches such as checkpoint inhibitors, cancer vaccines, adaptive cell transfer, and cytokines [138–140]. There are also complications with conventional immunotherapy methods such as Colitis secondary to immunotherapy coupled with diarrhea, abdominal pain, nausea, and vomiting. However, research has led to advancements in immunotherapy and other novel approaches to address these limitations. Subsequently, novel approaches to GC treatment are also being discussed [141–144].

4.1.1 Immune checkpoint inhibitors (ICIs)

T cells combat cancer by recognizing antigenic peptides presented on the Human Leukocyte Antigen (HLA) through T-cell receptor (TCR). This process is called immune surveillance and prevents tumor development. TSA is a specific target antigen for TCR on tumor cells. When the immune system becomes "blind" to TSA, tumors can grow uncontrollably, a phenomenon known as "tumor escape". Immune checkpoints serve as intrinsic components of the immune system, responsible for moderating the strength of immune responses to prevent harm to healthy cells. They come into play when proteins on T cells' surface, recognize and interact with partner proteins on other cells, including certain tumor cells. These partner proteins, known as immune checkpoint proteins, trigger an "off" signal upon binding with the checkpoint proteins, thereby dampening the immune response and preventing the destruction of cancer cells [139]. Immunotherapy drugs known as immune checkpoint inhibitors function by obstructing the binding of checkpoint proteins with their partners, thus thwarting the transmission of the off signal. Consequently, this enables T cells to target and eliminate cancer cells more effectively. Upon encountering cancer cells, cytotoxic T lymphocytes (CTLs) release interferon (IFN)-γ. Following its release, IFN-γ binds to IFN-γ receptors (IFN-γR) present on the surface of tumor cells. This interaction triggers the activation of the JAK-STAT signaling pathway, resulting in the increased expression of programmed death ligand-1 (PD-L1). Subsequently, when PD-1 receptors are blocked, inhibitory signals are transmitted to T cells, impairing their capacity to eradicate tumor cells (**Figure 5**) [146, 147]. PD-1 is significantly upregulated in thymocytes, NK cells, myeloid dendritic cells, and B and T cells. During inflammatory conditions, PD-L1 and 2 form functional interactions with PD-1 to protect normal tissues. However, this mechanism simultaneously enables tumors to evade immune detection. Therefore, anti-PD-1 agents showed the potential to restore T-cell activation by disrupting this interaction. mAbs targeting ICIs, like PD-1 and its corresponding ligand, have shown significant improvements in extending survival rates across different types of cancers, including advanced GC [148]. Nivolumab and Pembrolizumab are human mAbs of the IgG4 class, specifically engineered to block the PD-1 pathway (See **Table 3**). CTLA-4 is another critical immune checkpoint molecule found on the surface of T cells. This molecule interacts closely with CD28 and serves a crucial role in downregulating T-cell activation. The CTLA-4 pathway acts in an inhibitory role similar to that of PD-1, when bound by B7–1/2 on an APC [140]. This prevents T cells from binding to the CD28 receptor which is a co-stimulatory molecule on the surface of CD4 cells [151]. Thereby it facilitates the immune escape of tumors.

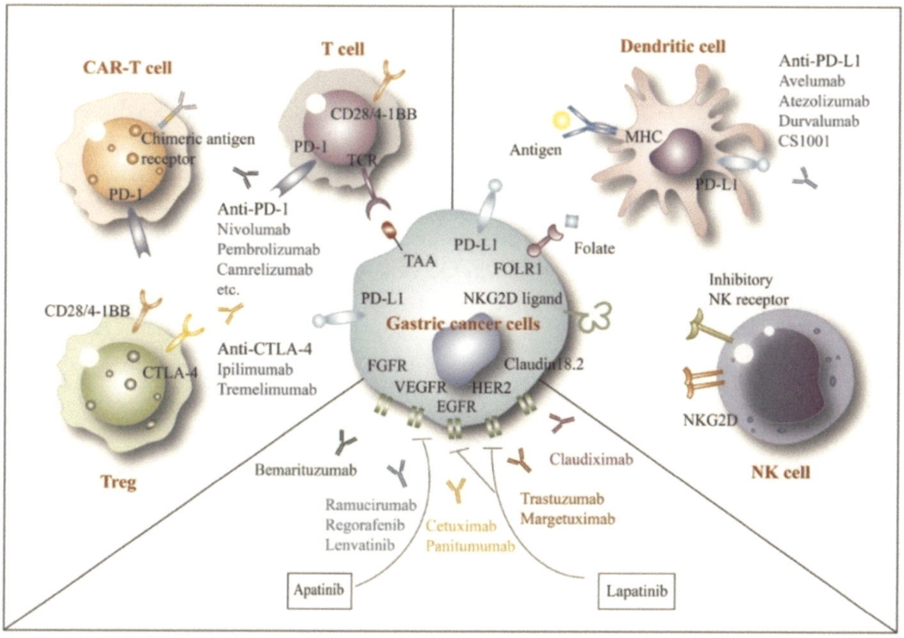

Figure 5.
Targets and immune checkpoints for GC [145]. Copyright 2021 Elsevier.

Study	Treatment line/Phase	Primary endpoint	Regimen	DCR/ ORR/ (%)
KEYNOTE-059	≥ 3rd line/ II	OS and PFS in PD-L1CPS ≥ 1	Pembrolizumab	–/57.1
KEYNOTE-061	2nd line/ III	OS and PFS in PD-L1CPS ≥ 1	Pembrolizumab	–/46.7
KEYNOTE-062	1st line/ III	OS and PFS in PD-L1CPS ≥ 1	CT + Pembrolizumab	–/64.7
KEYNOTE-164	≥ 2nd line/ II	ORR	Pembrolizumab	57/33
KEYNOTE-177	1st line/ III	PFS and OS	200 mg every 3 weeks	64.7/ 43.8
CheckMate-142	1st line/ II	ORR	CT	84/69
CheckMate-649	1st line/ III	PS and PFS in PD-L1 CPS ≥ 5	Nivolumab 3 mg/kg every 2 weeks plus ipilimumab 1 mg/kg every 6 weeks	–/70

DCR (disease control rate); PFS (progression-free survival); ORR (objective response rate); CT (chemotherapy).

Table 3.
Summarized overview of ongoing trials of checkpoint inhibitor drugs [149, 150].

4.1.1.1 CTLA-4 inhibitors

Antibodies targeting CTLA-4 bind specifically to these small molecules and alleviate T-cell suppression. Key examples approved of anti-CTLA-4 antibodies are

Tremelimumab and ipilimumab (**Table 3**). Ipilimumab obtained FDA approval in 2011 for the management of advanced melanoma. In a clinical study, Ipilimumab showed an objective response rate of 14% in patients with advanced gastric cancer. However, in another trial, Ipilimumab did not increase survival rates when employed as maintenance therapy following first-line chemotherapy for advanced GC or gastroesophageal junction cancer. T Tremelimumab, which acts as a specific CTLA-4 inhibitor is an IgG2 monoclonal human antibody that augments T-cell functionality. In a trial, Tremelimumab administered as a subsequent therapeutic approach showed a median PFS of 1.7 months and a median OS of 7.7 months in patients diagnosed with gastric cancer or gastroesophageal junction cancer following chemotherapy [145, 152, 153].

4.1.1.2 PD-1/PD-L1 inhibitors

Pembrolizumab and Nivolumab have been studied as potential treatments for advanced gastric cancer. In 2017, pembrolizumab was given approval by the Food and Drug Administration (FDA) as a third-line treatment for patients with positive CPS for PD-L1. Nivolumab showed significant survival rate enhancement and received approval as a third-line treatment for GC in Japan. Avelumab did not show significant improvement in overall survival when used as a maintenance and monotherapy treatment following first-line chemotherapy for advanced GC or gastric junction cancer. Overall, PD-1/PD-L1 inhibitors demonstrate clinical effectiveness in the management of advanced GC or gastroesophageal junction cancer., However, the benefits of monotherapy are relatively modest, particularly in later lines of treatment. Despite the approval of anti-PD-1 and PD-L1 therapies as monotherapies and in later lines of treatment, it is not likely that they will emerge as first-line therapies for GC [145, 154, 155].

4.1.1.3 Combinational therapy of Anti CTLA-4 and PD-1

The combination of anti-CTLA-4 and anti-PD-1 antibodies led to the inhibition of epithelial-mesenchymal transition (EMT) and reduced migration and invasion; a notable suppression of cell proliferation and apoptosis induction in MGC-803 and MKN-45 cells. Results from western blot analysis exhibited that this combination reduced the activation of β-catenin, MAPK, and PI3K/AKT signaling pathways. Additionally, *in vivo*, studies demonstrated that the combination therapy effectively inhibited tumor formation. Furthermore, transfection with si-PD-1 and si-CTLA resulted in significantly decreased levels of CTLA-4 and PD-1 in transcript levels. These findings suggest promising outcomes for the mentioned combination therapy in GC, yet further investigations are required (**Table 4**) [160].

4.1.2 Cellular immunotherapy

The utilization of immune cells as therapeutic interventions for cancer is referred to as cellular immunotherapy. T lymphocytes and NK cells cultivated in vitro are pivotal elements of these therapeutic strategies. These cells can undergo genetic modification to express certain T cell receptors (TCR-T immunotherapy) or chimeric antigen receptors (CAR-T Cell therapy) against desired targets [145].

Drugs(mAb)	Target therapies	VEGFR-2	Ramucirumab
			Apatinib
			Regorafenib
			Lenvatinib
		HER-2	Trastuzumab
			Margetuximab
	ICIs	PD-1	Camrelizumab (SHR-1210)
			Sintilimab
			Nivolumab
			Pembrolizumab
			Toripalimab (ISO01)
			Tislelizumab
		PD-L1	Avelumab
			Atezolizumab
			Durvalumab
			Sugemalimab (CS1001)
		CTLA-4	Tremelimumab
			Ipilimumab

Table 4.
mAb for targeted treatment of GC by inhibiting cell surface receptors [145, 156–159].

4.1.2.1 NK cell transfer therapy

NK cells indeed hold a pivotal role in combating tumor cells by hindering the inception and advancement of tumors (Section 1.2.2) [30]. They induce cytotoxicity by release of granzyme and perforin, antibody-dependent cytotoxicity (ADCC), secretion of TNF-α and IFN-γ, and induction of apoptosis through FAS/FASL and TRAIL/TRAILR complex interactions and modulate immune response. However, malignant cells develop mechanisms to evade immune responses. Moreover, NK cells' quantity and functionality decline as GC advances. Consequently, rectifying NK cell dysfunction may present a promising therapeutic avenue for GC. NK cell adoptive therapy presents a promising therapeutic avenue for gastric cancer. A Phase I clinical trial validated the safety and tolerability of autologous expanded NK cell therapy, which indicates the potential for effective combination treatment with other agents [161, 162].

4.1.2.2 CAR-T cell therapies

Targeted T-cell immunotherapy is the most thoroughly investigated and promising therapeutic pathway in the realm of GC. They have shown impressive results in clinical studies, particularly within hematological malignancies. These cells are genetically engineered to attack cancerous cells. A specific single-chain variable fragment (scFv) binding to a cancerous cell target is essential to engineering CAR-T cells. T cells are subsequently genetically engineered to express a chimeric receptor specifically designed to recognize and attack tumor cells (**Figure 5**) [163, 164]. Claudin18.2 is a membrane protein specific to the stomach. This molecule has been identified as a promising target in therapeutic approaches in GC as well as other types of cancer. CAR-T cells targeted towards this molecule eradicated gastric tumors in mice without causing unspecific toxicity. The latest clinical findings on GC and pancreatic cancer utilizing CAR-Claudin18.2 T cells have shown promise with a 33.3% overall objective response rate [165, 166]. NK group 2, member D (NKG2D) ligand AKA stress-induced ligand (NKG2DL) is a potential target for GC therapies. This molecule is typically expressed in GC cell lines. NKG2D-CAR-T cells, generated through the modification of CAR-T cells using second-generation CAR vectors, exhibit remarkable anti-tumor efficacy in both animal models and laboratory investigations [167]. HER2 molecule is an abnormally over-expressed molecule in 10–20% of GCs. HER2-CAR-T cells have demonstrated significant and persistent anti-tumor effects against GC cells in laboratory and animal models [168, 169]. Folate receptor 1 (FOLR1) serves as a target molecule that is prominently found overexpressed on the cell surface in more than 30% of GC patients, However, its expression in normal tissue is uncommon. This unique characteristic positions it as a promising target for CAR-T immunotherapy [170]. Prostate stem cell antigen (PSCA), is recognized for its glycosylphosphatidylinositol (GPI) anchored cell surface protein nature and presents as another target for CAR-T cell therapy in GC [171]. Mesothelin (MSLN) has also been considered a cellular target for CAR-T therapy in treating GC. Third-generation CAR-T cells (M28z10T) developed to specifically target MSLN, showed potent anti-tumor activity, underscoring their potential as a promising therapeutic strategy for GC [172].

4.1.2.3 TCR-T immunotherapy

This strategy involves the insertion of TCR genes targeting tumor antigens into the circulating T cells of patients, representing a modified form of adoptive T cell-based cancer immunotherapy. Encouraging outcomes have been observed with this approach across a spectrum of solid tumor types, including multiple myeloma, lung cancer, and synovial sarcoma [173–175]. Kita-Kyushu Lung Cancer Antigen-1 (KK-LC-1) is frequently identified as a cancer germline antigen in various epithelial cancers, including non-small cell lung cancer, triple-negative breast cancer, cervical cancer, and GC [176, 177]. CT83 expression is remarkably high in GC, and tumor lines positive for CT83 may be recognized by genetically modified T cells with the KK-LC-1 TCR (KK-LC-1 TCR-Ts) in vitro [178]. Another target for TCR-T therapy is potentially the New York esophageal squamous cell carcinoma 1 (NY-ESO-1). Its discovery is rooted in its ability to elicit detectable antibody responses in cancer patients. It is notable that following surgery, those without relapses had sustained reductions in or eradication of the serum levels of NY-ESO-1 antibodies [179]. These results demonstrated the KK-LC-1 TCR-Ts' encouraging potential for treating GC.

4.1.3 Vaccine treatment

Cancer therapeutic vaccines fall under the umbrella of active immunotherapy, designed to provoke a focused immune reaction against tumor antigens [180]. Peptides, DC, autologous tumor cells, and genetically engineered vaccines are among the vaccines used against cancer. A study evaluated the therapeutic potential of combining adjuvant immunotherapy with chemotherapy in GC patients, employing autologous tumor-derived Gp96 immunization considering that tumor antigens were the initial focus of tumor vaccination research [181]. In the group receiving the vaccine, patients exhibited enhanced rates of disease-free survival and 2-year OS compared to those undergoing chemotherapy alone, standing at 81.9% versus 67.9%. Another investigation, which focused on 9 individuals with advanced GC treated using the HER2/DC vaccine, documented partial clinical remission in a single patient, coupled with a decline in tumor marker levels such as CEA and CA19–9. Furthermore, there were observable anti-tumor effects observed in patients with advanced GC administered Melanoma-associated antigen A3 peptide (MAGE-A3)/DC [182].

Reportedly, 85% of diagnosed GC patients exhibit expression of Lymphocyte antigen 6 complex locus K (LY6K). In six patients with advanced GC, a Phase I clinical trial that investigated the vaccinations with LY6K-derived peptide showed that three out of 6 had more stable disease states and one had a 20% reduction in the size of metastases in their liver [183].

5. Nanomedicine and targeted therapies

Nanomedicine is a crucial tool in cancer management. Nanoparticles (NPs) can enhance the effectiveness of anticancer agents or function as anticancer agents themselves, targeting tumor cells in both active and inactive states based on the tumor type and TME conditions. This overcomes traditional cancer therapy limitations [184].

Polymeric NPs are used as carriers for chemotherapeutic drugs, due to their unique structures that encapsulate drug molecules. They address the limitations associated with these drugs such as instability, low solubility, toxicity, and poor permeability, improving cancer treatment outcomes [185, 186]. Numerous studies have explored the use of polymeric NPs (NPs) loaded with chemotherapeutic drugs like paclitaxel (PCT), doxorubicin (DOX), docetaxel (DCT), 5-fluorouracil (5FU), and other drugs for the treatment of GC. Recently, there has been increasing interest in hybrid drug delivery, which involves delivering two or more chemotherapeutic agents simultaneously, despite their delivery to the tumor site. This approach holds promise as a potent strategy to enhance GC treatment efficacy. However, the most significant challenge remains to achieve a more precise and targeted delivery of drug agents to the tumors' site, even with NPs. This difficulty arises from the varied physicochemical properties of anticancer agents. For example, researchers have developed NPs based on polyethylene glycol and poly(lactide-co-glycolide) (PEG-PLGA), loaded with 5-fluorouracil (SN-38-5FU@NPs) and irinotecan (SN-38), using the nanoprecipitation technique to improve the effectiveness of GC treatment [187–189]. Dendritic polymers like Poly(amidoamine) have potential for biomedical applications. PEGylated dendrimers with celastrol are used in GC therapy [184, 190]. Exosomes are nanoscale vesicles that range from 30 to 150 nanometers in diameter. They are secreted by various cell types and hold significant promise as GC therapy. Recent studies shed light on the role and outcome of exosome application in treating GC cell lines. Exosomes have potential as biomarkers for GC diagnosis and as targets for therapeutic approaches [191, 192]. Liposomes are colloidal vesicles made of phospholipids that mimic natural cell membranes. They have a high drug-loading capacity and can deliver hydrophilic and hydrophobic compounds. Liposomes are biodegradable, biocompatible, non-immunogenic, and non-toxic. They are widely used for delivering anticancer drugs in GC treatment [193, 194].

Metallic NPs are used as novel anticancer agents in the treatment of GC. They are produced by capping and reducing metal precursors like zinc acetate dihydrate, copper nitrate, gold halides, and silver nitrate [195]. Metallic NPs can be used alone or with other drugs to achieve better anticancer effects against GC. Silver, gold, nickel oxide, zinc oxide, and cobalt oxide NPs have shown outstanding outcomes against GC cells by augmenting targeting precision, facilitating controlled drug release, supporting imaging modalities, and enhancing gene modification mechanisms [196]. Gold NPs have shown potential as a versatile tool for both diagnosing and treating cancer. Studies have found them to be effective against GC cells while demonstrating good biocompatibility, In AGS cell lines, inhibiting autophagy-related pathways and up-regulating apoptotic signaling [197, 198]. Silver NPs synthesized using eco-friendly methods and natural sources have been shown to significantly inhibit the proliferation of gastric cancer (GC) cells, including the AGS and MNK45 cell lines. This inhibition is achieved by inducing apoptosis, which suggests a promising approach for effective GC therapy [184]. Additionally, nickel oxide and cobalt NPs synthesized through chemical methods displayed cytotoxicity against AGS-GC cell lines in a dose-dependent manner. Nevertheless, nickel oxide and cobalt NPs both exhibited minimal toxicity towards normal fibroblast cells (L929) [197, 198].

5.1 Theranostic NPs

Theranostic NPs are sophisticated nanosystems, that facilitate highly accurate and individualized disease management by amalgamating diagnostic and therapeutic functionality (**Figure 6**) [200]. Superparamagnetic iron oxide nanoparticles (SPIONs) can be used for magnetic resonance imaging (MRI), while gold

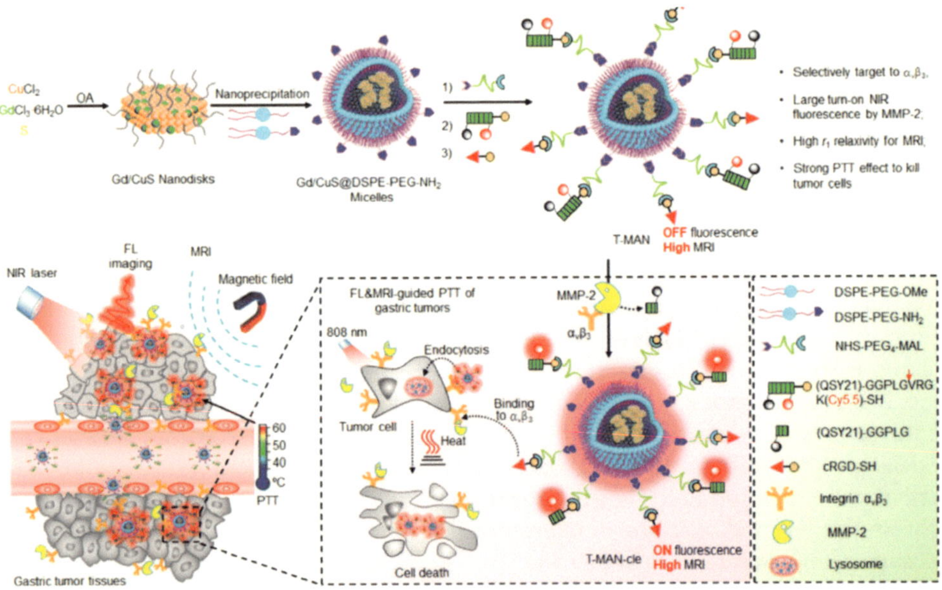

Figure 6.
The diagram depicts NPs designed for gastric cancer theranostics. Specifically, it showcases a tumor-targeted and matrix metalloprotease-2 (MMP-2)-activatable nanoprobe (T-MAN). This nanoprobe is developed by modifying Gd-doped CuS micellar NPs with cRGD, covalently. This modification allows for selective entry and accumulation of the nanoprobe in gastric tumors via αvβ3 integrin-mediated active delivery [199]. Copyright 2019 American Chemical Society.

Nanoparticles	Theranostic		Ref.
	Therapeutic strategy	Imaging strategy	
ICG-loaded lactosome	PTT	Fluorescence	[202]
Carbon–gold hybrid NPs	PTT	Fluorescence	[203]
RGD-CuS-Cy5.5 NPs	PTT	CT/MRI	[204, 205]
W18O49 NPs	PTT	CT/ fluorescence	[204, 206]
PEGPCL-IR780-MET NPs	PTT	PA/ fluorescence	[206, 207]
Hyaluronidase-sensitive mesoporous silica NPs	PDT	Fluorescence	[207, 208]
Ternary copper-based chalcogenide nano platform CuS–NiS2 nanomaterials	PTT/PDT	MRI	[209]
Folic acid–sericin–cholesterol/IR780 micelles	PTT/PDT	Fluorescence	[201, 210]
DOX-IR820 NPs	PTT/chemotherapy	Fluorescence	[211]
IR820/paclitaxel/imiquimod/encapsulated thermosensitive liposome	PTT/PDT/chemotherapy	Fluorescence	[201, 212]
PTX-R837-IR820@TSL	PTT/PDT/chemotherapy/ Immunotherapy	Fluorescence	[207]
Cisplatin/ICG loaded PLGA-(DSPE-PEG2000) NPs	Chemotherapy	Fluorescence	[212, 213]
Chlorin e6 functionalized silk fibroin NPs	Chemotherapy	Fluorescence	[208, 210]
Oxaliplatin-Au-Fe3O4-Herceptin NPs	Chemotherapy	MRI	[205, 213]

Photothermal therapy (PTT); Photodynamic therapy (PDT); Arginine-Glycine-Aspartic (RGD).

Table 5.
Nanotechnology-based theranostic(therapeutic/diagnostic) agents for GC.

nanoparticles (NPs) are well-suited for computed tomography (CT). Therefore, they are commonly used in the construction of theranostic systems. Additionally, some photosensitizers, such as chlorin e6 and IR780, have both tumor-toxic and imaging abilities. This is because they can absorb near-infrared (NIR) light to induce fluorescence and generate reactive oxygen species (ROS) and/or heat [201]. though the structure and assembly of these nano-based theranostic systems can be complex, many have already been reported, demonstrating their potential in treating gastric cancer (refer to **Table 5**) [200, 214].

Xin Luo and et.al developed a nanocarrier system that enhances siRNA delivery using a PD-L1 knock-down system. The system involved creating disulfide-polyethylene glycol-folic acid-conjugated polyethyleneimine coupled with Fe3O4 SPIONs. This approach entailed encapsulating FA-PEG-SS-PEI and SPIONs utilizing a ligand-exchange method, followed by combining this combination with cationic micelles complexed with synthesized siRNA. The product underwent characterization and exhibited excellent contrast for T2-weighted cancer MRI using cellular MRI. PD-L1 siRNAs exhibited notable knock-down of PD-L1, supporting their use as a theranostic approach [215, 216].

6. Other treatments

A notable therapeutic approach involves oncolytic viruses, which possess the ability to selectively destroy tumor cells while leaving healthy cells unharmed [217]. By causing the lysis of tumor cells, oncolytic viruses release TANs as well as tumor-associated antigens, thereby triggering a specific immune response. Rigvir, H101, and T-VEC are among the primary oncolytic viruses utilized in cancer therapy, with Rigvir being the pioneering oncolytic virus approved for clinical use [218].

Employing cytokines and non-specific immune boosters, which can be administered either before or concurrently with antigens to improve the immune response or modify its characteristics without inducing an antigenic response, represents an alternative approach for treating GC. Among these non-specific immune boosters, cytokines and lentinan are commonly employed in clinical settings. Lentinan, a β-1,3-D-glucan, is clinically employed as an immunomodulatory medication for tumor treatment [145].

Combination therapies are often used to achieve better treatment outcomes. For example, combining chemotherapy and trastuzumab in a clinical trial resulted in significantly longer OS rates. Gene therapy in combination with anti-cancer drugs presents a promising opportunity to enhance treatment outcomes [219]. An aptamer-siRNA chimera combined with 5-fluorouracil (5-FU) in a collagen membrane can specifically bind to GC cells, delivering 5-FU to the affected site while suppressing drug-resistant genes [220].

7. Conclusion and outlook

Gastric cancer (GC) is one of the prevalent cancers with poor prognosis. GC is responsible for a significant number of cancer-related deaths across the globe, particularly in its advanced stages (median survival of less than 1 year for metastatic patients). GC is known as a heterogeneous cancer, Furthermore, the biological differences between tumors in Eastern and Western countries have made finding a standard treatment that can include all types of GCs challenging. GC is a multifactorial disease caused by genetic and epigenetic factors; All these factors affect the biological regulatory processes of the cell such as proliferation, differentiation, and cell metabolism. In addition, tumor microenvironment (TEM) in GC differs from normal tissue regarding metabolism. These modifications include the shift from aerobic respiration to glycolysis which leads to lactate production and acidification of the TEM. The TEM contains a diverse range of cells, such as cancer cells, CAFs, pericytes, and other immune cells, and has irregular vasculature. Additionally, it is subject to various mutations. The conditions that were mentioned earlier have led to a lack of response to traditional forms of treatment like surgery, endoscopy, chemotherapy, and radiation therapy. The current treatment methods and the combined treatment of these methods, due to the resistance to the treatment, do not have the necessary effectiveness and are even associated with various side effects; Consequently, new treatment methods with biological approaches are felt more and more as a basic need to develop new treatment strategies. Studying tumor microenvironments and the interplay between cancer cells and immune cells has spurred the development of novel immunotherapy strategies, including the utilization of nanoparticles. A variety of immunotherapies including immune checkpoint inhibitors (CTLA-4 inhibitors, PD-1/PD-L1 inhibitors and

Combinational therapy of Anti CTLA-4 and PD-1), cellular immunotherapy (NK cell transfer, TCR-T immunotherapy, and CAR-T cell therapies), cytokines and vaccine therapy have shown promising effects results against GC. NPs are utilized to actively target the tumor site. Moreover, morphological changes in the tumor TEM, such as variations in pH levels and distinct properties of its vessel wall, enable NPs to passively target cancer cells. Further, the usage of theranostic NPs, a combination of therapy and diagnosis, enables better monitoring of response during treatment. These capabilities allow NPs to effectively overcome limitations in GC therapy.

Despite the significant advancements made in the last decade, there are still many challenges to achieving a fully effective method with minimal side effects for the treatment of GC; including reducing the side effects caused by immunotherapy (colitis secondary to immunotherapy with diarrhea, abdominal pain, nausea), toxicity of nanomaterials, etc. In fact, it seems that we cannot eliminate conventional treatment methods, especially surgery and chemotherapy, anytime soon. In the near future, more efforts will be made to fully identify various biological regulatory factors such as ferroptosis, immunological GC, more effective factors on TEM, genomic data of different molecular subtypes, nanomaterials with appropriate biocompatibility and biodegradability. Additionally, scientists will be working to identify reliable predictive factors for early detection which will promise more effective treatment methods.

Author contributions

All authors contributed to the study conception, design, material preparation, data collection, and analysis. The first draft of the manuscript was written by and all authors commented on previous versions of the manuscript. All authors read and approved the final manuscript.

Author details

Pegah Mousavi[1], Ali Ahmadi[2], Shakila Behzadifar[3], Javad Mohammadnejad[3] and Seyed Mohammad Hosseini[4*]

1 Immunology Research Center, Tabriz University of Medical Sciences, Tabriz, Iran

2 Department of Medical Biotechnologies and Translational Medicine, University of Milan, Italy

3 Department of Life Science Engineering Faculty of Modern Science and Technology, Nano Biotechnology Group, University of Tehran, Iran

4 Department of Medical Nanotechnology, Faculty of Advanced Technologies in Medicine, Iran University of Medical Sciences, Tehran, Iran

*Address all correspondence to: hosseini.semo@iums.ac.ir

References

[1] Januszewicz W, Turkot MH, Malfertheiner P, Regula J. A global perspective on gastric cancer screening: Which concepts are feasible, and when? Cancers. 2023;**15**(3):664

[2] López MJ et al. Characteristics of gastric cancer around the world. Critical Reviews in Oncology/Hematology. 2023; **181**:103841

[3] Ajani JA et al. Gastric cancer, version 2.2022, NCCN clinical practice guidelines in oncology. Journal of the National Comprehensive Cancer Network. 2022;**20**(2):167-192

[4] Charalampakis N et al. Trimodality treatment in gastric and gastroesophageal junction cancers: Current approach and future perspectives. World Journal of Gastrointestinal Oncology. 2022;**14**(1): 181

[5] Jia Z et al. Positive *H. Pylori* status predicts better prognosis of non-cardiac gastric cancer patients: Results from cohort study and meta-analysis. BMC Cancer. 2022;**22**(1):155

[6] Shin J, Park YS. Unusual or uncommon histology of gastric cancer. Journal of Gastric Cancer. 2024;**24**(1):69

[7] Rawla P, Barsouk A. Epidemiology of gastric cancer: Global trends, risk factors and prevention. Gastroenterology Review/Przegląd Gastroenterologiczny. 2019;**14**(1):26-38

[8] Mukaisho K, Nakayama T, Hagiwara T, Hattori T, Sugihara H. Two distinct etiologies of gastric cardia adenocarcinoma: Interactions among pH, *Helicobacter pylori*, and bile acids. Frontiers in Microbiology. 2015;**6**:412

[9] Zhang Y et al. Healthy lifestyle counteracts the risk effect of genetic factors on incident gout: A large population-based longitudinal study. BMC Medicine. 2022;**20**(1):138

[10] Sastre J, García-Saenz JA, Díaz-Rubio E. Chemotherapy for gastric cancer. World Journal of Gastroenterology: WJG. 2006;**12**(2):204

[11] Högner A, Moehler M. Immunotherapy in gastric cancer. Current Oncology. 2022;**29**(3): 1559-1574

[12] Amjad MT, Chidharla A, Kasi A. Cancer chemotherapy. In: StatPearls. Treasure Island (FL): StatPearls Publishing; 2023. PMID: 33232037

[13] Matsueda S, Graham DY. Immunotherapy in gastric cancer. World Journal of Gastroenterology: WJG. 2014; **20**(7):1657

[14] Sah B et al. Post-operative complications of gastric cancer surgery: Female gender at high risk. European Journal of Cancer Care. 2009;**18**(2): 202-208

[15] Gao C, Liu F, Ye Q, Guo A. Cancer-associated fibroblasts affect tumor metabolism and immune microenvironment in gastric cancer and identification of its characteristic genes. Journal of Oncology. 2023;**2023**:1424589

[16] Yan Y, Wang LF, Wang RF. Role of cancer-associated fibroblasts in invasion and metastasis of gastric cancer. World Journal of Gastroenterology. 2015; **21**(33):9717-9726

[17] Sun H, Wang X, Wang X, Xu M, Sheng W. The role of cancer-associated fibroblasts in tumorigenesis of gastric

cancer. Cell Death & Disease. 2022; **13**(10):874

[18] Cirri P, Chiarugi P. Cancer associated fibroblasts: The dark side of the coin. American Journal of Cancer Research. 2011;**1**(4):482-497

[19] Hanahan D, Coussens LM. Accessories to the crime: Functions of cells recruited to the tumor microenvironment. Cancer Cell. 2012;**21**(3):309-322

[20] Erez N, Truitt M, Olson P, Arron ST, Hanahan D. Cancer-associated fibroblasts are activated in incipient neoplasia to orchestrate tumor-promoting inflammation in an NF-kappaB-dependent manner. Cancer Cell. 2010;**17**(2):135-147

[21] Yamauchi M, Gibbons DL, Zong C, Fradette JJ, Bota-Rabassedas N, Kurie JM. Fibroblast heterogeneity and its impact on extracellular matrix and immune landscape remodeling in cancer. Matrix Biology. 2020;**91-92**:8-18

[22] Mao X et al. Crosstalk between cancer-associated fibroblasts and immune cells in the tumor microenvironment: New findings and future perspectives. Molecular Cancer. 2021;**20**(1):131

[23] Kumar V et al. Single-cell atlas of lineage states, tumor microenvironment, and subtype-specific expression programs in gastric cancer. Cancer Discovery. 2022;**12**(3):670-691

[24] Li X et al. Single-cell RNA sequencing reveals a pro-invasive cancer-associated fibroblast subgroup associated with poor clinical outcomes in patients with gastric cancer. Theranostics. 2022;**12**(2):620-638

[25] Zhao Z, Mak TK, Shi Y, Li K, Huo M, Zhang C. Integrative analysis of cancer-associated fibroblast signature in gastric cancer. Heliyon. 2023;**9**(9):e19217

[26] Rogers S et al. Cancer-associated fibroblasts influence Wnt/PCP signaling in gastric cancer cells by cytoneme-based dissemination of ROR2. Proceedings of the National Academy of Sciences of the United States of America. 2023;**120**(39): e2217612120

[27] Kharaishvili G, Simkova D, Bouchalova K, Gachechiladze M, Narsia N, Bouchal J. The role of cancer-associated fibroblasts, solid stress and other microenvironmental factors in tumor progression and therapy resistance. Cancer Cell International. 2014;**14**:41

[28] Sammarco G et al. Mast cells, angiogenesis and Lymphangiogenesis in human gastric cancer. International Journal of Molecular Sciences. 2019; **20**(9)

[29] Xu X et al. Immunology and immunotherapy in gastric cancer. Clinical and Experimental Medicine. 2023;**23**(7):3189-3204

[30] Zhao Y, Bai Y, Shen M, Li Y. Therapeutic strategies for gastric cancer targeting immune cells: Future directions. Frontiers in Immunology. 2022;**13**:992762

[31] Yang J, Liu X, Cheng Y, Zhang J, Ji F, Ling Z. Roles of plasmacytoid dendritic cells in gastric cancer. Frontiers in Oncology. 2022;**12**:818314

[32] Chang WJ, Du Y, Zhao X, Ma LY, Cao GW. Inflammation-related factors predicting prognosis of gastric cancer. World Journal of Gastroenterology. 2014;**20**(16):4586-4596

[33] Wolf NK, Kissiov DU, Raulet DH. Roles of natural killer cells in immunity

to cancer, and applications to immunotherapy. Nature Reviews. Immunology. 2023;**23**(2):90-105

[34] Wu SY, Fu T, Jiang YZ, Shao ZM. Natural killer cells in cancer biology and therapy. Molecular Cancer. 2020;**19**(1): 120

[35] Fuertes MB, Domaica CI, Zwirner NW. Leveraging NKG2D ligands in Immuno-oncology. Frontiers in Immunology. 2021;**12**:713158

[36] Devillier R, Chrétien AS, Pagliardini T, Salem N, Blaise D, Olive D. Mechanisms of NK cell dysfunction in the tumor microenvironment and current clinical approaches to harness NK cell potential for immunotherapy. Journal of Leukocyte Biology. 2021;**109**(6): 1071-1088

[37] Hu Z, Xu X, Wei H. The adverse impact of tumor microenvironment on NK-cell. Frontiers in Immunology. 2021; **12**:633361

[38] van Vliet AA, Georgoudaki AM, Raimo M, de Gruijl TD, Spanholtz J. Adoptive NK cell therapy: A promising treatment Prospect for metastatic melanoma. Cancers (Basel). 2021;**13**(18)

[39] Engström A, Erlandsson A, Delbro D, Wijkander J. Conditioned media from macrophages of M1, but not M2 phenotype, inhibit the proliferation of the colon cancer cell lines HT-29 and CACO-2. International Journal of Oncology. 2014;**44**(2):385-392

[40] Arango Duque G, Descoteaux A. Macrophage cytokines: Involvement in immunity and infectious diseases. Frontiers in Immunology. 2014;**5**:491

[41] Kurahara H et al. Significance of M2-polarized tumor-associated macrophage in pancreatic cancer. The Journal of Surgical Research. 2011;**167**(2):e211-e219

[42] Li W et al. Gastric cancer-derived mesenchymal stromal cells trigger M2 macrophage polarization that promotes metastasis and EMT in gastric cancer. Cell Death & Disease. 2019;**10**(12):918

[43] Kaparakis M et al. Macrophages are mediators of gastritis in acute *Helicobacter pylori* infection in C57BL/6 mice. Infection and Immunity. 2008; **76**(5):2235-2239

[44] Sathe A et al. Single-cell genomic characterization reveals the cellular reprogramming of the gastric tumor microenvironment. Clinical Cancer Research. 2020;**26**(11):2640-2653

[45] Eissmann MF et al. IL-33-mediated mast cell activation promotes gastric cancer through macrophage mobilization. Nature Communications. 2019;**10**(1):2735

[46] Lin C et al. Tumour-associated macrophages-derived CXCL8 determines immune evasion through autonomous PD-L1 expression in gastric cancer. Gut. 2019;**68**(10):1764-1773

[47] Zhou Z et al. A C-X-C chemokine receptor type 2-dominated cross-talk between tumor cells and macrophages drives gastric cancer metastasis. Clinical Cancer Research. 2019;**25**(11):3317-3328

[48] Li S et al. Tumor-associated neutrophils induce EMT by IL-17a to promote migration and invasion in gastric cancer cells. Journal of Experimental & Clinical Cancer Research. 2019;**38**(1):6

[49] Wang TT et al. Tumour-activated neutrophils in gastric cancer foster immune suppression and disease

progression through GM-CSF-PD-L1 pathway. Gut. 2017;**66**(11):1900-1911

[50] Coffelt SB, Wellenstein MD, de Visser KE. Neutrophils in cancer: neutral no more. Nature Reviews. Cancer. 2016; **16**(7):431-446

[51] Mao Z et al. CXCL5 promotes gastric cancer metastasis by inducing epithelial-mesenchymal transition and activating neutrophils. Oncogene. 2020;**9**(7):63

[52] Zhang W et al. Interaction with neutrophils promotes gastric cancer cell migration and invasion by inducing epithelial-mesenchymal transition. Oncology Reports. 2017;**38**(5):2959-2966

[53] Law AMK, Valdes-Mora F, Gallego-Ortega D. Myeloid-derived suppressor cells as a therapeutic target for cancer. Cells. 2020;**9**(3)

[54] Bayik D, Lee J, Lathia JD. The role of myeloid-derived suppressor cells in tumor growth and metastasis. Experientia Supplementum. 2022;**113**: 189-217

[55] Wang L, Chang EW, Wong SC, Ong SM, Chong DQ, Ling KL. Increased myeloid-derived suppressor cells in gastric cancer correlate with cancer stage and plasma S100A8/A9 proinflammatory proteins. Journal of Immunology. 2013;**190**(2):794-804

[56] Cui C, Lan P, Fu L. The role of myeloid-derived suppressor cells in gastrointestinal cancer. Cancer Communications (London). 2021;**41**(6): 442-471

[57] Chen X et al. Accumulation of T-helper 22 cells, interleukin-22 and myeloid-derived suppressor cells promotes gastric cancer progression in elderly patients. Oncology Letters. 2018; **16**(1):253-261

[58] Moaaz M, Lotfy H, Elsherbini B, Motawea MA, Fadali G. TGF-β enhances the anti-inflammatory effect of tumor-infiltrating CD33+11b+HLA-DR myeloid-derived suppressor cells in gastric cancer: A possible relation to MicroRNA-494. Asian Pacific Journal of Cancer Prevention. 2020;**21**(11): 3393-3403

[59] Wang PF et al. Prognostic role of pretreatment circulating MDSCs in patients with solid malignancies: A meta-analysis of 40 studies. Oncoimmunology. 2018;**7**(10):e1494113

[60] Shen P, Fillatreau S. Antibody-independent functions of B cells: A focus on cytokines. Nature Reviews. Immunology. 2015;**15**(7):441-451

[61] Sarvaria A, Madrigal JA, Saudemont A. B cell regulation in cancer and anti-tumor immunity. Cellular & Molecular Immunology. 2017;**14**(8): 662-674

[62] van der Leun AM, Thommen DS, Schumacher TN. CD8(+) T cell states in human cancer: Insights from single-cell analysis. Nature Reviews. Cancer. 2020; **20**(4):218-232

[63] Basu A et al. Differentiation and regulation of T(H) cells: A balancing act for cancer immunotherapy. Frontiers in Immunology. 2021;**12**: 669474

[64] Kang BW, Kim JG, Lee IH, Bae HI, Seo AN. Clinical significance of tumor-infiltrating lymphocytes for gastric cancer in the era of immunology. World Journal of Gastrointestinal Oncology. 2017;**9**(7):293

[65] Nagase H et al. ICOS(+) Foxp3(+) TILs in gastric cancer are prognostic markers and effector regulatory T cells associated with *Helicobacter pylori*.

International Journal of Cancer. 2017; **140**(3):686-695

[66] Miyara M et al. Functional delineation and differentiation dynamics of human CD4+ T cells expressing the FoxP3 transcription factor. Immunity. 2009;**30**(6):899-911

[67] Salama P et al. Tumor-infiltrating FOXP3+ T regulatory cells show strong prognostic significance in colorectal cancer. Journal of Clinical Oncology. 2009;**27**(2):186-192

[68] Okita Y et al. Role of tumor-infiltrating CD11b+ antigen-presenting cells in the progression of gastric cancer. Journal of Surgical Research. 2014; **186**(1):192-200

[69] Takeuchi H, Maehara Y, Tokunaga E, Koga T, Kakeji Y, Sugimachi K. Prognostic significance of natural killer cell activity in patients with gastric carcinoma: A multivariate analysis. The American Journal of Gastroenterology. 2001;**96**(2):574-578

[70] Lee S-C et al. Phase I trial of expanded, activated autologous NK-cell infusions with trastuzumab in patients with HER2-positive cancers. Clinical Cancer Research. 2020;**26**(17): 4494-4502

[71] Ishigami S et al. Prognostic value of intratumoral natural killer cells in gastric carcinoma. Cancer. 2000;**88**(3):577-583

[72] Xie M-Z, Ding K, Tang Y-P, Hu B-L, Li K-Z, Li J-L, et al. Percentage of natural killer (NK) cells in peripheral blood is associated with prognosis in patients with gastric cancer: A retrospective study from a single center. Medical Science Monitor: International Medical Journal of Experimental and Clinical Research. 2021;**27**:e927464-e927461

[73] Guo Z, Zhou C, Zhou L, Wang Z, Zhu X, Mu X. Overexpression of DAPK1-mediated inhibition of IKKβ/CSN5/PD-L1 axis enhances natural killer cell killing ability and inhibits tumor immune evasion in gastric cancer. Cellular Immunology. 2022;**372**:104469

[74] Pernot S et al. Infiltrating and peripheral immune cell analysis in advanced gastric cancer according to the Lauren classification and its prognostic significance. Gastric Cancer. 2020;**23**: 73-81

[75] Fabian KP et al. PD-L1 targeting high-affinity NK (t-haNK) cells induce direct antitumor effects and target suppressive MDSC populations. Journal for Immunotherapy of Cancer. 2020; **8**(1)

[76] Yu S et al. Activated HIF1α of tumor cells promotes chemoresistance development via recruiting GDF15-producing tumor-associated macrophages in gastric cancer. Cancer Immunology, Immunotherapy. 2020;**69**: 1973-1987

[77] Lin C et al. Tumour-associated macrophages-derived CXCL8 determines immune evasion through autonomous PD-L1 expression in gastric cancer. Gut. 2019. DOI: 10.1136/gutjnl-2018-316324

[78] Peng L-S et al. Tumor-associated monocytes/macrophages impair NK-cell function via TGFβ1 in human gastric cancer. Cancer Immunology Research. 2017;**5**(3):248-256

[79] Wang H-C et al. Tumor-associated macrophages promote epigenetic silencing of gelsolin through DNA methyltransferase 1 in gastric cancer cells. Cancer Immunology Research. 2017;**5**(10):885-897

[80] Liu X et al. Poor clinical outcomes of intratumoral dendritic cell–specific intercellular adhesion molecule 3–grabbing non-integrin–positive macrophages associated with immune evasion in gastric cancer. European Journal of Cancer. 2020;**128**:27-37

[81] Jeremiasen M et al. Tumor-associated CD68+, CD163+, and MARCO + macrophages as prognostic biomarkers in patients with treatment-naïve gastroesophageal adenocarcinoma. Frontiers in Oncology. 2020;**10**:534761

[82] Zhang H et al. Poor clinical outcomes and immunoevasive contexture in intratumoral IL-10-producing macrophages enriched gastric cancer patients. Annals of Surgery. 2022;**275**(4): e626-e635

[83] Zhang X, Shi H, Yuan X, Jiang P, Qian H, Xu W. Tumor-derived exosomes induce N2 polarization of neutrophils to promote gastric cancer cell migration. Molecular Cancer. 2018; **17**(1):146

[84] Li TJ et al. Interleukin-17-producing neutrophils link inflammatory stimuli to disease progression by promoting angiogenesis in gastric cancer. Clinical Cancer Research. 2017;**23**(6):1575-1585

[85] Zhou X et al. PMN-MDSCs accumulation induced by CXCL1 promotes CD8+ T cells exhaustion in gastric cancer. Cancer Letters. 2022;**532**: 215598

[86] Thompson ED et al. Patterns of PD-L1 expression and CD8 T cell infiltration in gastric adenocarcinomas and associated immune stroma. Gut. 2016. gutjnl-2015-310839. DOI: 10.1016/j.canlet.2022.215598

[87] He X et al. Impact of intratumoural CD73 expression on prognosis and therapeutic response in patients with gastric cancer. European Journal of Cancer. 2021;**157**:114-123

[88] Wang J et al. Intratumoral CXCR5+ CD8+ T associates with favorable clinical outcomes and immunogenic contexture in gastric cancer. Nature Communications. 2021;**12**(1):3080

[89] Jin K et al. Poor clinical outcomes and immunoevasive contexture in CXCL13+ CD8+ T cells enriched gastric cancer patients. Oncoimmunology. 2021; **10**(1):1915560

[90] Nagase H et al. ICOS+ F oxp3+ TIL s in gastric cancer are prognostic markers and effector regulatory T cells associated with *Helicobacter pylori*. International Journal of Cancer. 2017;**140**(3):686-695

[91] Fei Y et al. Intratumoral Foxp3+ RORγt+ T cell infiltration determines poor prognosis and immunoevasive contexture in gastric cancer patients. Cancer Immunology, Immunotherapy. 2022;**71**(1):1-11

[92] Wang J et al. Tumor-infiltrating γδT cells predict prognosis and adjuvant chemotherapeutic benefit in patients with gastric cancer. Oncoimmunology. 2017;**6**(11):e1353858

[93] Lin R et al. Fatty acid oxidation controls CD8+ tissue-resident memory T-cell survival in gastric adenocarcinoma. Cancer Immunology Research. 2020;**8**(4):479-492

[94] Kwak Y et al. Differential prognostic impact of CD8+ T cells based on human leucocyte antigen I and PD-L1 expression in microsatellite-unstable gastric cancer. British Journal of Cancer. 2020;**122**(9):1399-1408

[95] Chen K et al. TIM3+ cells in gastric cancer: Clinical correlates and

association with immune context. British Journal of Cancer. 2022;**126**(1):100-108

[96] Qu Y et al. The effects of TNF-α/TNFR2 in regulatory T cells on the microenvironment and progression of gastric cancer. International Journal of Cancer. 2022;**150**(8):1373-1391

[97] Zhu F et al. Ring finger protein 31–mediated atypical ubiquitination stabilizes forkhead box P3 and thereby stimulates regulatory T-cell function. Journal of Biological Chemistry. 2018; **293**(52):20099-20111

[98] Mao F-Y et al. Increased tumor-infiltrating CD45RA−CCR7−regulatory T-cell subset with immunosuppressive properties foster gastric cancer progress. Cell Death & Disease. 2017;**8**(8):e3002

[99] Kindlund B et al. CD4+ regulatory T cells in gastric cancer mucosa are proliferating and express high levels of IL-10 but little TGF-β. Gastric Cancer. 2017;**20**:116-125

[100] Liu X et al. Regulatory T cells and M2 macrophages present diverse prognostic value in gastric cancer patients with different clinicopathologic characteristics and chemotherapy strategies. Journal of Translational Medicine. 2019;**17**(1):1-11

[101] Ni Z et al. Tumor-infiltrating B cell is associated with the control of progression of gastric cancer. Immunologic Research. 2021;**69**:43-52

[102] Ji L et al. Blockade of β-catenin-induced CCL28 suppresses gastric cancer progression via inhibition of Treg cell infiltration. Cancer Research. 2020; **80**(10):2004-2016

[103] Fang H et al. Intratumoral interleukin-9 delineates a distinct immunogenic class of gastric cancer patients with better prognosis and adjuvant chemotherapeutic response. Oncoimmunology. 2020;**9**(1):1856468

[104] Sun L et al. Human gastric cancer mesenchymal stem cell-derived IL15 contributes to tumor cell epithelial-mesenchymal transition via upregulation Tregs ratio and PD-1 expression in CD4 (+)T cell. Stem Cells and Development. 2018;**27**(17):1203-1214

[105] Wang JT et al. Intratumoral IL17-producing cells infiltration correlate with antitumor immune contexture and improved response to adjuvant chemotherapy in gastric cancer. Annals of Oncology. 2019;**30**(2):266-273

[106] Bie Q et al. IL-17B/IL-17RB signaling cascade contributes to self-renewal and tumorigenesis of cancer stem cells by regulating Beclin-1 ubiquitination. Oncogene. 2021;**40**(12): 2200-2216

[107] Wu P et al. Adaptive mechanisms of tumor therapy resistance driven by tumor microenvironment. Frontiers in Cell and Developmental Biology. 2021;**9**: 641469

[108] Subhash VV, Yeo MS, Tan WL, Yong WP. Strategies and advancements in harnessing the immune system for gastric cancer immunotherapy. Journal of Immunology Research, vol. 2015;**2015**

[109] Pettersen EO et al. Targeting tumour hypoxia to prevent cancer metastasis. From biology, biosensing and technology to drug development: The METOXIA consortium. Journal of Enzyme Inhibition and Medicinal Chemistry. 2015;**30**(5):689-721

[110] Al Tameemi W, Dale TP, Al-Jumaily RMK, Forsyth NR. Hypoxia-modified cancer cell metabolism.

Frontiers in Cell and Developmental Biology. 2019;7:4

[111] Das V, Štěpánková J, Hajdúch M, Miller JH. Role of tumor hypoxia in acquisition of resistance to microtubule-stabilizing drugs. Biochimica et Biophysica Acta (BBA)-Reviews on Cancer. 2015;**1855**(2):172-182

[112] Li M, Li G, Yang X, Yin W, Lv G, Wang S. HIF in gastric cancer: Regulation and therapeutic target. Molecules. 2022;**27**(15):4893

[113] Griffiths EA, Pritchard S, Welch I, Price PM, West C. Is the hypoxia-inducible factor pathway important in gastric cancer? European Journal of Cancer. 2005;**41**(18): 2792-2805

[114] Xuan Y, Wang YN. Hypoxia/IL-1α axis promotes gastric cancer progression and drug resistance. Journal of Digestive Diseases. 2017;**18**(9):511-520

[115] Sun X et al. Hypoxia-mediated cancer stem cell resistance and targeted therapy. Biomedicine & Pharmacotherapy. 2020;**130**:110623

[116] Kang BW, Chau I. Current status and future potential of predictive biomarkers for immune checkpoint inhibitors in gastric cancer. ESMO Open. 2020;**5**(4):e000791

[117] Liu Y et al. Signaling pathways of oxidative stress response: The potential therapeutic targets in gastric cancer. Frontiers in Immunology. 2023;**14**: 1139589

[118] Gu H et al. Reactive oxygen species-mediated tumor microenvironment transformation: The mechanism of radioresistant gastric cancer. Oxidative Medicine and Cellular Longevity. 2018; **2018**

[119] Allegra A, Murdaca G, Mirabile G, Gangemi S. Redox Signaling modulates activity of immune checkpoint inhibitors in cancer patients. Biomedicine. 2023; **11**(5):1325

[120] Aboelella NS, Brandle C, Kim T, Ding Z-C, Zhou G. Oxidative stress in the tumor microenvironment and its relevance to cancer immunotherapy. Cancers. 2021;**13**(5):986

[121] Leone A, Roca MS, Ciardiello C, Costantini S, Budillon A. Oxidative stress gene expression profile correlates with cancer patient poor prognosis: Identification of crucial pathways might select novel therapeutic approaches. Oxidative Medicine and Cellular Longevity. 2017;**2017**

[122] Justus CR, Sanderlin EJ, Yang LV. Molecular connections between cancer cell metabolism and the tumor microenvironment. International Journal of Molecular Sciences. 2015;**16**(5): 11055-11086

[123] Chiche J, Brahimi-Horn MC, Pouysségur J. Tumour hypoxia induces a metabolic shift causing acidosis: A common feature in cancer. Journal of Cellular and Molecular Medicine. 2010; **14**(4):771-794

[124] Wu H et al. T-cells produce acidic niches in lymph nodes to suppress their own effector functions. Nature Communications. 2020;**11**(1):4113

[125] Colombani T et al. Oxygen-generating cryogels restore T cell mediated cytotoxicity in hypoxic tumors. Advanced Functional Materials. 2021;**31**(37):2102234

[126] Ramello MC, Haura EB, Abate-Daga D. CAR-T cells and combination therapies: what's next in the immunotherapy revolution?

Pharmacological Research. 2018;**129**: 194-203

[127] Bai J, Gao Z, Li X, Dong L, Han W, Nie J. Regulation of PD-1/PD-L1 pathway and resistance to PD-1/PD-L1 blockade. Oncotarget. 2017;**8**(66): 110693

[128] Wu Y, Chen W, Xu ZP, Gu W. PD-L1 distribution and perspective for cancer immunotherapy—Blockade, knockdown, or inhibition. Frontiers in Immunology. 2019;**10**:2022

[129] Petryszyn P, Chapelle N, Matysiak-Budnik T. Gastric cancer: Where are we heading? Digestive Diseases. 2020;**38**(4): 280-285

[130] Arn CR, Halla KJ, Gill S. Tisotumab Vedotin safety and tolerability in clinical practice: Managing adverse events. Journal of the Advanced Practitioner in Oncology. 2023;**14**(2):139

[131] Galata C, Ronellenfitsch U, Blank S, Reißfelder C, Hardt J. Postoperative morbidity and failure to rescue in surgery for gastric cancer: A single center retrospective cohort study of 1107 patients from 1972 to 2014. Cancers. 2020;**12**(7):1953

[132] Das M. Neoadjuvant chemotherapy: Survival benefit in gastric cancer. The Lancet Oncology. 2017;**18**(6):e307

[133] Maisey N, Norman A, Prior Y, Cunningham D. Chemotherapy for primary gastric lymphoma: Does in-patient observation prevent complications? Clinical Oncology. 2004; **16**(1):48-52

[134] Natale JJ. Overview of the prevention and management of CINV. The American Journal of Managed Care. 2018;**24**(18 Suppl.):S391-S397

[135] Andreyev HJN, Davidson SE, Gillespie C, Allum WH, Swarbrick E. Practice guidance on the management of acute and chronic gastrointestinal problems arising as a result of treatment for cancer. Gut. 2011. gutjnl-2011-300563. DOI: 10.1016/S1470-2045(17)30321-2

[136] Ng SP, Leong T. Role of radiation therapy in gastric cancer. Annals of Surgical Oncology. 2021;**28**(8):4151-4157

[137] Kennedy GD, Heise CP. Radiation colitis and proctitis. Clinics in Colon and Rectal Surgery. 2007;**20**(01):064-072

[138] Riley RS, June CH, Langer R, Mitchell MJ. Delivery technologies for cancer immunotherapy. Nature Reviews Drug Discovery. 2019;**18**(3):175-196

[139] Zhao Q et al. Immunotherapy for gastric cancer: Dilemmas and prospect. Briefings in Functional Genomics. 2019; **18**(2):107-112

[140] Grierson P, Lim K-H, Amin M. Immunotherapy in gastrointestinal cancers. Journal of Gastrointestinal Oncology. 2017;**8**(3):474

[141] De Velasco G et al. Comprehensive meta-analysis of key immune-related adverse events from CTLA-4 and PD-1/PD-L1 inhibitors in cancer patients. Cancer Immunology Research. 2017; **5**(4):312-318

[142] Larkin J et al. Combined nivolumab and ipilimumab or monotherapy in untreated melanoma. New England Journal of Medicine. 2015;**373**(1):23-34

[143] Marthey L et al. Cancer immunotherapy with anti-CTLA-4 monoclonal antibodies induces an inflammatory bowel disease. Journal of Crohn's and Colitis. 2016;**10**(4):395-401

[144] Akkanapally V, Bai X-F, Basu S. Therapeutic immunomodulation in gastric cancer. Cancers. 2024;**16**(3):560

[145] Li K, Zhang A, Li X, Zhang H, Zhao L. Advances in clinical immunotherapy for gastric cancer. Biochimica et Biophysica Acta (BBA)-Reviews on Cancer. 2021;**1876**(2):188615

[146] Chen L, Han X. Anti–PD-1/PD-L1 therapy of human cancer: Past, present, and future. The Journal of Clinical Investigation. 2015;**125**(9):3384-3391

[147] Park J-J et al. B7-H1/CD80 interaction is required for the induction and maintenance of peripheral T-cell tolerance. Blood, The Journal of the American Society of Hematology. 2010; **116**(8):1291-1298

[148] Takei S, Kawazoe A, Shitara K. The new era of immunotherapy in gastric cancer. Cancers. 2022;**14**(4):1054

[149] Miljanic M, Capasso A, Triplett TA, Eckhardt SG, Aung KL. Immune checkpoint blockade in gastrointestinal cancers: The current status and emerging paradigms. Journal of Immunotherapy and Precision Oncology. 2020;**3**(1):3-15

[150] Shimozaki K, Nakayama I, Hirota T, Yamaguchi K. Current strategy to treat immunogenic gastrointestinal cancers: Perspectives for a new era. Cells. 2023;**12**(7):1049

[151] Sznol M, Melero I. Revisiting anti-CTLA-4 antibodies in combination with PD-1 blockade for cancer immunotherapy. Annals of Oncology. 2021;**32**(3):295-297

[152] Janjigian YY et al. CheckMate-032: Phase I/II, open-label study of safety and activity of nivolumab (nivo) alone or with ipilimumab (ipi) in advanced and metastatic (A/M) gastric cancer (GC). Biochimica et Biophysica Acta (BBA) - Reviews on Cancer. 2016;**1876**(2):188615

[153] Kelly RJ et al. Safety and efficacy of durvalumab and tremelimumab alone or in combination in patients with advanced gastric and gastroesophageal junction adenocarcinoma. Clinical Cancer Research. 2020;**26**(4):846-854

[154] Shitara K et al. Pembrolizumab versus paclitaxel for previously treated, advanced gastric or gastro-oesophageal junction cancer (KEYNOTE-061): A randomised, open-label, controlled, phase 3 trial. The Lancet. 2018; **392**(10142):123-133

[155] Moehler M et al. Phase III trial of avelumab maintenance after first-line induction chemotherapy versus continuation of chemotherapy in patients with gastric cancers: Results from JAVELIN gastric 100. Journal of Clinical Oncology. 2021;**39**(9):966

[156] Li K, Zhang A, Li X, Zhang H, Zhao L. Advances in clinical immunotherapy for gastric cancer. Biochimica et Biophysica Acta (BBA) - Reviews on Cancer. 2021;**1876**(2):188615

[157] Yu Y et al. Changes in expression of multiple checkpoint molecules and infiltration of tumor immune cells after neoadjuvant chemotherapy in gastric cancer. Journal of Cancer. 2019;**10**(12): 2754

[158] Muro K et al. Pembrolizumab for patients with PD-L1-positive advanced gastric cancer (KEYNOTE-012): A multicentre, open-label, phase 1b trial. The Lancet Oncology. 2016;**17**(6):717-726

[159] Kang Y-K et al. Nivolumab in patients with advanced gastric or gastro-oesophageal junction cancer refractory to, or intolerant of, at least two previous chemotherapy regimens (ONO-4538-12,

ATTRACTION-2): A randomised, double-blind, placebo-controlled, phase 3 trial. The Lancet. 2017;**390**(10111): 2461-2471

[160] Wang B, Qin L, Ren M, Sun H. Effects of combination of anti-CTLA-4 and anti-PD-1 on gastric cancer cells proliferation, apoptosis and metastasis. Cellular Physiology and Biochemistry. 2018;**49**(1):260-270

[161] Du Y, Wei Y. Therapeutic potential of natural killer cells in gastric cancer. Frontiers in Immunology. 2019;**9**:3095

[162] Sakamoto N et al. Phase I clinical trial of autologous NK cell therapy using novel expansion method in patients with advanced digestive cancer. Journal of Translational Medicine. 2015;**13**:1-13

[163] Alcantara M, Du Rusquec P, Romano E. Current clinical evidence and potential solutions to increase benefit of CAR T-cell therapy for patients with solid tumors. Oncoimmunology. 2020; **9**(1):1777064

[164] Bębnowska D et al. CAR-T cell therapy—An overview of targets in gastric cancer. Journal of Clinical Medicine. 2020;**9**(6):1894

[165] Zhan X et al. Phase I trial of Claudin 18.2-specific chimeric antigen receptor T cells for advanced gastric and pancreatic adenocarcinoma. Journal of Translational Medicine. 2019;**13**(1):277

[166] Jiang H et al. Claudin18. 2-specific chimeric antigen receptor engineered T cells for the treatment of gastric cancer. JNCI: Journal of the National Cancer Institute. 2019;**111**(4):409-418

[167] Tao K et al. Development of NKG2D-based chimeric antigen receptor-T cells for gastric cancer treatment. Cancer Chemotherapy and Pharmacology. 2018;**82**:815-827

[168] Grillo F, Fassan M, Sarocchi F, Fiocca R, Mastracci L. HER2 heterogeneity in gastric/ gastroesophageal cancers: From benchside to practice. World Journal of Gastroenterology. 2016;**22**(26):5879

[169] Song Y et al. Effective and persistent antitumor activity of HER2-directed CAR-T cells against gastric cancer cells in vitro and xenotransplanted tumors in vivo. Protein & Cell. 2018;**9**(10): 867-878

[170] Kim M et al. Folate receptor 1 (FOLR1) targeted chimeric antigen receptor (CAR) T cells for the treatment of gastric cancer. PLoS One. 2018;**13**(6): e0198347

[171] Maude SL et al. Tisagenlecleucel in children and young adults with B-cell lymphoblastic leukemia. New England Journal of Medicine. 2018;**378**(5): 439-448

[172] Lv J et al. Mesothelin is a target of chimeric antigen receptor T cells for treating gastric cancer. Journal of Hematology & Oncology. 2019;**12**(1): 1-14

[173] Jahn L et al. TCR-based therapy for multiple myeloma and other B-cell malignancies targeting intracellular transcription factor BOB1. Blood. 2017; **129**(10):1284-1295

[174] Robbins PF et al. A pilot trial using lymphocytes genetically engineered with an NY-ESO-1-reactive T-cell receptor: Long-term follow-up and correlates with response. Clinical Cancer Research. 2015;**21**(5):1019-1027

[175] Xia Y et al. Treatment of metastatic non-small cell lung cancer with NY-ESO-1

specific TCR engineered-T cells in a phase I clinical trial: A case report. Oncology Letters. 2018;**16**(6):6998-7007

[176] Ichiki Y et al. Development of adoptive immunotherapy with KK-LC-1-specific TCR-transduced γδT cells against lung cancer cells. Cancer Science. 2020;**111**(11):4021-4030

[177] Shida A et al. Cancer/testis antigen, Kita-Kyushu lung cancer antigen-1 and ABCD stratification for diagnosing gastric cancers. World Journal of Gastroenterology. 2020;**26**(4):424-432

[178] Marcinkowski B et al. Cancer targeting by TCR gene-engineered T cells directed against Kita-Kyushu lung cancer Antigen-1. Journal for Immunotherapy of Cancer (MDPI). 2019;7(1):229

[179] Fujiwara S et al. NY-ESO-1 antibody as a novel tumour marker of gastric cancer. British Journal of Cancer. 2013;**108**(5):1119-1125

[180] Watson HA et al. L-selectin enhanced T cells improve the efficacy of cancer immunotherapy. Frontiers in Immunology. 2019;**10**:1321

[181] Zhang K et al. Phase II trial of adjuvant immunotherapy with autologous tumor-derived Gp96 vaccination in patients with gastric cancer. Journal of Cancer. 2017;**8**(10):1826-1832

[182] Subklewe M, von Bergwelt-Baildon M, Humpe A. Chimeric antigen receptor T cells: A race to revolutionize cancer therapy. Transfusion Medicine and Hemotherapy. 2019;**46**(1):15-24

[183] Ishikawa H et al. Phase I clinical trial of vaccination with LY6K-derived peptide in patients with advanced gastric cancer. Gastric Cancer. 2014;**17**(1):173-180

[184] Hani U et al. Novel drug delivery systems as an emerging platform for stomach cancer therapy. Pharmaceutics. 2022;**14**(8):1576

[185] Zielińska A et al. Polymeric nanoparticles: Production, characterization, toxicology and ecotoxicology. Molecules. 2020;**25**(16)

[186] Hosseini S, Mohammadnejad J, Salamat S, Zadeh ZB, Tanhaei M, Ramakrishna S. Theranostic polymeric nanoparticles as a new approach in cancer therapy and diagnosis: A review. Materials Today Chemistry. 2023;**29**:101400

[187] Suriya Prabha A, Dorothy R, Jancirani S, Rajendran S, Singh G, Senthil Kumaran S. In: Nanotoxicity S, Rajendran A, Mukherjee TA, Nguyen CG, Shukla RK, editors. Chapter 7 - Recent Advances in the Study of Toxicity of Polymer-Based Nanomaterials. Elsevier; 2020. pp. 143-165

[188] Hong J, Feng Z. Synergic fabrication of combination therapy of irinotecan and 5-fluorouracil encapsulated polymeric nanoparticles for the treatment of gastric cancer therapy. Process Biochemistry. 2021;**106**:191-198

[189] Narmani A et al. Biomedical applications of PLGA nanoparticles in nanomedicine: Advances in drug delivery systems and cancer therapy. Expert Opinion on Drug Delivery. no. just-accepted. 2023

[190] Hosseini SM, Mohammadnejad J, Yousefnia H, Alirezapour B, Rezayan AH. Development of 177Lu-Cetuximab-PAMAM dendrimeric

nanosystem: A novel theranostic radioimmunoconjugate. Journal of Cancer Research and Clinical Oncology. 2023;**149**(10):7779-7791

[191] Pan L et al. Exosomes-mediated transfer of long noncoding RNA ZFAS1 promotes gastric cancer progression. Journal of Cancer Research and Clinical Oncology. 2017;**143**(6):991-1004

[192] Fu M, Gu J, Jiang P, Qian H, Xu W, Zhang X. Exosomes in gastric cancer: Roles, mechanisms, and applications. Molecular Cancer. 2019;**18**: 1-12

[193] Das M, Huang L. Liposomal nanostructures for drug delivery in gastrointestinal cancers. Journal of Pharmacology and Experimental Therapeutics. 2019;**370**(3):647-656

[194] Pattni BS, Chupin VV, Torchilin VP. New developments in liposomal drug delivery. Chemical Reviews. 2015;**115**(19):10938-10966

[195] Sharma A, Goyal AK, Rath G. Recent advances in metal nanoparticles in cancer therapy. Journal of Drug Targeting. 2018;**26**(8):617-632

[196] Salapa J, Bushman A, Lowe K, Irudayaraj J. Nano drug delivery systems in upper gastrointestinal cancer therapy. Nano Convergence. 2020;7(1): 1-17

[197] Hosseinkhah M et al. Cytotoxic potential of nickel oxide nanoparticles functionalized with glutamic acid and conjugated with thiosemicarbazide (NiO@ Glu/TSC) against human gastric cancer cells. Journal of Cluster Science. 2022;**33**(5):2045-2053

[198] Jarestan M et al. Preparation, characterization, and anticancer efficacy of novel cobalt oxide nanoparticles conjugated with thiosemicarbazide. 3 Biotech. 2020;**10**:1-9

[199] Shi H et al. Magnetic semiconductor Gd-doping CuS nanoparticles as Activatable Nanoprobes for bimodal imaging and targeted Photothermal therapy of gastric Tumors. Nano Letters. 2019;**19**(2):937-947

[200] Hosseini SM, Mohammadnejad J, Najafi-Taher R, Zadeh ZB, Tanhaei M, Ramakrishna S. Multifunctional carbon-based nanoparticles: Theranostic applications in cancer therapy and diagnosis. ACS Applied Bio Materials. 2023;**6**(4):1323-1338

[201] Deng L, Guo W, Li G, Hu Y, Zhang L-M. Hydrophobic IR780 loaded sericin nanomicelles for phototherapy with enhanced antitumor efficiency. International Journal of Pharmaceutics. 2019;**566**:549-556

[202] Tsujimoto H et al. Theranostic photosensitive nanoparticles for lymph node metastasis of gastric cancer. Annals of Surgical Oncology. 2015;**22**(3): 923-928

[203] Zhang A et al. Carbon-gold hybrid nanoprobes for real-time imaging, photothermal/photodynamic and nanozyme oxidative therapy. Theranostics. 2019;**9**(12):3443

[204] Shi H et al. Tumor-targeting CuS nanoparticles for multimodal imaging and guided photothermal therapy of lymph node metastasis. Acta Biomaterialia. 2018;**72**:256-265

[205] Liu D et al. Target-specific delivery of oxaliplatin to HER2-positive gastric cancer cells in vivo using oxaliplatin-au-fe3o4-herceptin nanoparticles. Oncology Letters. 2018; **15**(5):8079-8087

[206] Yang Z et al. Tumor-targeting W18O49 nanoparticles for dual-modality imaging and guided heat-shock-response-inhibited photothermal therapy in gastric cancer. Particle & Particle Systems Characterization. 2019; **36**(7):1900124

[207] Yang Z et al. Defeating relapsed and refractory malignancies through a nano-enabled mitochondria-mediated respiratory inhibition and damage pathway. Biomaterials. 2020;**229**:119580

[208] Yao H, Xu K, Zhou J, Zhou L, Wei S. A tumor microenvironment destroyer for efficient cancer suppression. ACS Biomaterials Science & Engineering. 2019;**6**(1):450-462

[209] Chen J et al. CuS–NiS2 nanomaterials for MRI guided phototherapy of gastric carcinoma via triggering mitochondria-mediated apoptosis and MLKL/CAPG-mediated necroptosis. Nanotoxicology. 2020;**14**(6):774-787

[210] Abtab SMT et al. Reticular chemistry in action: A hydrolytically stable MOF capturing twice its weight in adsorbed water. Chem. 2018;**4**(1):94-105

[211] Zhou Y, Sun X, Zhou L, Zhang X. pH-sensitive and long-circulation nanoparticles for near-infrared fluorescence imaging-monitored and chemo-photothermal synergistic treatment against gastric cancer. Frontiers in Pharmacology. 2020;**11**:610883

[212] Meng X et al. Photothermal/photodynamic therapy with immune-adjuvant liposomal complexes for effective gastric cancer therapy. Particle & Particle Systems Characterization. 2019;**36**(6):1900015

[213] Shi T et al. Enhanced legumain-recognition and NIR controlled released of cisplatin-indocyanine nanosphere against gastric carcinoma. European Journal of Pharmacology. 2017;**794**:184-192

[214] Li X, Ai S, Lu X, Liu S, Guan W. Nanotechnology-based strategies for gastric cancer imaging and treatment. RSC Advances. 2021;**11**(56):35392-35407

[215] Arshad R et al. Novel perspectives towards RNA-based nano-theranostic approaches for cancer management. Nanomaterials. 2021;**11**(12):3330

[216] Luo X, Peng X, Hou J, Wu S, Shen J, Wang L. Folic acid-functionalized polyethylenimine superparamagnetic iron oxide nanoparticles as theranostic agents for magnetic resonance imaging and PD-L1 siRNA delivery for gastric cancer. International Journal of Nanomedicine. 2017;**11**:5331-5343

[217] Ahmadi A, Ghaleh HE, Dorostkar R, Farzanehpour M, Bolandian M. Oncolytic Coxsackievirus and the mechanisms of its effects on cancer: A narrative review. Current Cancer Therapy Reviews. 2021;**17**(3):173-178

[218] Chen L, Zuo M, Zhou Q, Wang Y. Oncolytic virotherapy in cancer treatment: Challenges and optimization prospects. Frontiers in Immunology. 2023;**14**:1308890

[219] Dai X, Tan C. Combination of microRNA therapeutics with small-molecule anticancer drugs: Mechanism of action and co-delivery nanocarriers. Advanced Drug Delivery Reviews. 2015; **81**:184-197

[220] Chen W et al. Construction of Aptamer-siRNA chimera/PEI/5-FU/carbon nanotube/collagen membranes for the treatment of peritoneal dissemination of drug-resistant gastric cancer. Advanced Healthcare Materials. 2020;**9**(21):2001153